Much of this Book was Previously Published in "The Drinker's Woman." (Still, a hundred pages or so is new stuff!)

DOES HE DRINK TOO MUCH?

By Beth Copeland, M.A., LMHC
(Formerly writing as Ariel I.)

Copyright Mary Copeland 2014

Printed by CreateSpace-Amazon
Applied Psychology Publishing, LLC
Jacksonville, FL USA

"The need for change bulldozed a road down the center of my mind."

By--Maya Angelou

Table of Contents

Introduction

Chapter 1
What's Really Going on With Him? 1

Chapter 2
Bad Behavior? Let Us Count the Ways 49

Chapter 3
Relationships Problems: 95
What's Different about Yours?

Chapter 4
Did You See the Switch? 125
From Handsome Prince to Horse's Butt?

Chapter 5
Wanna Know How Bad 155
His Drinking Problem Really Is?

Chapter 6
Denial: Who's He Fooling? 191

Chapter 7
Prince Being Beastly; How Fares 211
Our Fair Princess?

Chapter 8
Making A New Plan!
The Proper Care of a Princess 253

Chapter 9
Are You Safe? 307

Introduction

Does he drink too much?
You may ask: But how much is too much?
That's a very good question.

We define "too much" drinking as "drinking enough to cause problems in his life and/or the lives of those close to him." *That's* too much.

Whether it's only one beer or a case of Jim Beam, you can diagnose problem drinking when the changes it causes begin causing life and people problems. Almost all drinkers's women talk first about what he drinks and how much, but that approach misses the mark. (Any over-drinker worth his salt easily hides most of whatever he's doing; all that you know is not the whole story.) But No! It's not what he drinks, or how much—it's what happens when he drinks that counts.

Want to know precisely how bad his drinking really is? You're going to find out in Chapter 5. Before that, some interesting information.

Let's sit ourselves down for a little talk, a talk about him and his drinking, a talk about what his drinking has caused in his behavior and what it's doing to you.

First, we'll talk about how you've been dealing with it. Here's a little story to start our conversation.

I was raised on old-fashioned Southern cooking. For at least two hundred years before me, my ancestors lived on the same, delicious, old-fashioned Southern cooking.

For those of you who don't know real Southern cooking, the kind you get on poor homesteads, where vegetables are plentiful but money scarce, I'll tell you a bit about it. Genuine Southern cooking incorporates great dollops of lard (a fancy word for pig fat, which includes saved bacon drippings, lots of bacon drippings, Yum! The old-fashioned Southern cook uses lard for every form of oil in cooking. We use it in everything. Fried chicken. Biscuits. Vegetables. Custards, cornbread, and cakes.

As I entered my 50s, physicians occasionally inquired about my diet (likely because my cholesterol flopped way over the line). I told them what I cooked and ate and, to show off that I knew about healthy eating, always added that I ate lots of vegetables (leaving out the fact that they are cooked to near puree, and soaked in pig fat).

On one of these occasions, my primary insisted we discuss my diet yet again. Yet again I told her that I was working on cutting down on pork, roasts and hams and ribs and chops. And butter. (I wanted to show off that I was smart about cholesterol.)

"I eat a lot of poultry and fish," I added, (leaving out that they were deep-fried in lard flavored heavily with bacon drippings). I'd add, "not much red meat, " (a phrase I picked up from a pamphlet in her office that I thought would impress her. But she sat, listening while staring into my file. "Beth, I see here that all of your listed ancestors have died of heart attacks or strokes," she said. "Yep," I answered, proud because our family didn't have other disorders (as if it were a personal accomplishment).

She laid down my file and looked into my eyes. "If your standard diet follows the Old Southern way, you know, with buckets of lard and bacon drippings, I can't help but wonder if that could be what has killed them, and certainly killed them before their time." Then she just sat there.

I (perceptively) felt she wanted me to respond, but it took me a moment to parse what she had said. "Does she want me to give up lard?" I wondered

Can't do that. Nothin' in the world does biscuits and pie crusts and cornbread to die for like lard with bacon drippings.

I knew right then she must be from up north, at least north Georgia (gone all big city), and she just didn't know any better. Besides, I liked her, so I didn't ask her if she had lost her mind.)

"Well, I could try cutting down on fat in my food," I said, knowing that my family wouldn't stand for it. And no one would come to my house for dinner anymore! Why, fried fish and chicken and French fries aren't even edible unless cooked with bacon drippings—might as well serve them raw. What about in our vegetables and soups? (All this was an issue at the time because I was between rotten husbands; finding a new mate was a prime objective. But with that kind of cooking, what man would have me?) I was flustered.

After a pause where I just didn't know what to say, she said, "Oh, well, it's your life, and your funeral." She closed my file and walked to the door, where she turned and added brightly, "Oh, let me tell you something that may come in handy. I just read that Walmart and Costco now sell cut-rate caskets. You might want to note that for your children's information." Then she left the office.

Oh, how I wanted to say something to sound clever, intelligent, but I couldn't. Likely because I wasn't.

Begrudgingly, my children's destinies weighing on me, I did start making small changes in my diet and my cooking, with the family complaining all the way about how my cooking had gone bad. But I persisted, for their sake more than mine. And we all benefitted.

Today, after the years it took to completely change, I eat mostly vegetables, fresh, often raw. Not one ounce of lard has entered my kitchen in years and years (which *may* be related to my weight and cholesterol improvements).

I began asking people I knew (except family, heaven forbid) about how they cooked and ate in a healthy way. I especially stayed on the lookout for any who were cutting down on lard, side meat, and such. Some had helpful hints to share, but not one has ever had any info on how to crisp pork skins without lard.

I bought a couple of "healthy" cookbooks and, surprisingly to me, began to enjoy both the new way of cooking and the food. I like science and early on began to think of my cooking as science experiments.

I also bought herbs and seasonings (looking for one that tastes like bacon grease but I never found any). Shortly, I set out a small herb garden and today I still take great pleasure in it.

Now, to move into the point of this story requires another story:

Progressing in my trial-and-error research cooking, I brewed up a pot of potato soup. Having added everything the recipe called for but it still tasted like something was missing, I remembered that one of my books said that rosemary was especially good in soups. I went out the back door to pick some. I wasn't at all sure about how much was needed and remembered that my Granny said that when you are unsure of how much of a vegetable to pick, you should pick about a handful for each serving you expect to be eaten.

That advice had always worked for me, so I altered it slightly for how much fresh rosemary it should take. (I didn't pick a handful for every serving; I knew herbs taste stronger than other vegetables, so I pulled about a handful of the short needles for the whole pot of soup.)

Soon the soup was smelling good, but after cooling a spoonful to taste, I yelped and spit it out into a napkin. Phtoo-ey!

It was awful. I checked to see if I had spooned my soup out of the wrong pot, but no, it was the rosemary-potato soup. (I could tell by the crust of rosemary covering the top of it.)

Pause.

A few days later, I determined to try again. Let's pretend it was you in the chef's hat that day, though I know none of you has ever done anything so awful in the kitchen. Here's my question to all you smart gals (and any woman looking for answers is smart): Would you use the same methods that didn't work now the next time you made potato soup?

No? Why not?

Right! Because *experience* proved that way didn't work!

This time you would do something different! I'm heartened to hear that. You're saying that you wouldn't keep on using a recipe technique that didn't work, that didn't give you the outcome you wanted. You're saying you would ditch that approach and find a better one. Most Excellent!

But I'll bet you have kept on using your same old tactics on your guy, the ones you've used in the past that haven't ever worked for you, trying the same or similar things to get your guy to "do right" over and over, and always getting the same results—none of them what you wanted. Oh, on the surface of it you may think some worked—he changed. For a while.

Here's how you can tell what worked: Did any changes he made last? That was a plan that worked.

Or did most slip away with things gradually drifting back to being dreadful? That was a plan that didn't work.

Recognizing that your tactics, how you responded to him when he didn't do right—your tactics, the fruit of your mighty mental labors, didn't work is a scary event. Yet, like so many things that appear scary from a distance, when you grabbed it by the horns, you saw it was a teddy bar disguised as a mastodon. You didn't want to see that your ways weren't working because you didn't know what else to do. Well, you're about to fill your whole bag with new tricks.

Your blaring signal that your tactics did not work to get him to do right need no longer be scary because you'll have a number of new, often easier, ways to deal with him.

It's tricky; sometimes it appeared he was going to go with the program, but it didn't last. But if they don't last, then they weren't really fixed. If you plug a leaky boat and the plug works initially, stopping the flow about to sink you, but shortly, the water begins seeping in around the plug, or the plug completely pops out, did you really fix it? Na-ah.

At best, in both cases, you got a short reprieve. Which is also a wonderful experience. But you wouldn't keep using a plug or a recipe that didn't work; why would you keep using a tactic for dealing with him and his shenanigans that hasn't ever worked?

And No! again—it's not because you're dumb! It's because you simply haven't known any better ways. Know how I know that? You would have used the better ways if you had known about them.

But now the cable on your flying trapeze is unraveling faster; to save yourself from sure disaster you need a fix that really works. Most often, when a commonsense fix doesn't work, you will find that you were mistaken about what the original problem actually was. In these cases, it requires finding and targeting the real problem. Rosemary is great, wonderful in soups, it's even has antibiotic properties! But using too much or too little, or fixing the wrong problem, either of these have likely plagued you.

But be assured, one of your major blocks until now has been that you've been firing all your magnificent arrows at the wrong targets. And that is only because you (and several hundred million other people in the United States) don't understand what is actually going wrong in over-drinking.

Here's your Very Good News: If your lack of success with changing your guy is because you haven't known any better ways to go about it—you're about to get a boatload of new ways. I promise you that as you practice these simple techniques, everything in your life is about to change.

Chapter 1

What's Really Going on With Him?

We both know why you're here: You wouldn't have picked up a book with this title if you were just looking for a rainy day read. Indeed, I fashioned it to pull a woman who is desperately seeking be ready for a new kind of help and guidance. And the guidance you seek is in a very specific category, a man's over-drinking. Be assured; I have some information for you that you haven't seen before. It will be new to you, and the techniques it teaches will work.

The first thing to discuss is this largely ignored fact: A man's drinking doesn't have to be "so bad" it's called alcoholism for everyone around him to be justified in getting desperate about changing him. Think back, to the earliest days when he started to change, to act differently or even bad when drinking, you were plopped into a worrisome and unpleasant bunch of situations, with concern and worry that over time has steadily worsened, increasingly pressing you, draining you. Then he, his behavior, began to wound you, leave you feeling adrift, and as if you were somehow in the wrong. You by now have spent countless hours and days trying to change him, and as many trying to change something about yourself (usually something he has said is awry, something he has blamed for sparking his bad behavior). You've had little or no success at any of this and have become increasingly unhappy.

Most books written about men who drink too much start by explaining that he's not a bad guy, then tell you that he just has an illness. Then they tell you that if you love him more and focus on him more and work harder (no matter how hateful or disgusting he has become), your new efforts will make it all get better.

Oh, happy day! They give you the power to change everything! Just what you were looking for! What you could do to fix it. Yay!

But think: In other words, other books put the burden on you! They give you instructions and most of them are do-able, and they do it with the assurance that your efforts can change him. Do this, do that, set up an intervention, mortgage your house to get him into treatment. And by all means, be more understanding, forgiving, loving, and compassionate.

Bull.

Worst of all, other books have the gall to tell you to do all those things as if they actually work!

Many of you have already discovered that they don't. At least their instructions didn't make the kind of changes that stayed changed. Even though it cost you a year's income.

You won't be getting any talk here about loving him better to make him better. Yet books that focus on your love for him as the key to his getting well sell really big though. I tell you this because their success with the women of over-drinkers proves one very important point. Their jumping off the shelves into desperate hands proves what I'm saying here about you, about who you really are. You are a lover and a giver. You are willing to give your all to help him and salvage your families.

To boot, you are very comfortable with feeling like it's all up to you, and in shouldering the weight of blame. Yes, you are the kind of person who feels responsibility for caring for others. It's a worthy ideal and surely the thinking of the loving Creator, but your instructors are only telling you part of the story. The true change will only be done by him. And for the few who finally make it, most of them have lost their women before they made that change.

For many women, all that would be enough to convince them the job can't be done by their efforts, but not you. That's because of who you are; no matter how much of a mess you can sometimes think you are, in fact you are incredibly good, strong, loving, giving, forgiving, and so much more.

Oh yes, you remember many of the wrongs and hurts, yet you fight on despite that. Want proof? Look at you—reading this book! Looking for help to get him to do right.

You're going to learn here exactly what's going on with him, especially in his steadily deteriorating mind-brain. You're going to finally understand his ever-worsening behavior, most especially the things he does and the things he says; you will understand your situation so well that you won't be easily knocked off your emotional pins anymore when he does some of the .yucky things he does.

(Note 1: One of the first things we will change is the way people think about any form of "treatment." The word "treatment" implies that one will get well if he will just takes it. With alcohol and other addiction treatment most people assume that is the case . Be informed: It is not!)
(Note 2: Making sure you know this is one major reason I wrote this book. Even if he goes to "treatment," he will not get well there! The best he can get at others's hands is a brief break in his addiction and the behavior it encourages. From there on, it's up to him—day by day, minute by minute, for the rest of his entire life—to put into practice huge, multiple new behaviors, including becoming willing to take advice!)

That last necessity is extremely difficult for over-drinkers; they have fought so long to convince the world that they are just fine and don't need help that they no longer remember any other way. The "habit" of refusing advice—lest others think they need help—doesn't leave easily.

Even if he does well after "treatment" (as only a handful will), establishing healthy sobriety, he still will never be okay, "well," over it. The brain cells he killed with alcohol will not grow back. The unhealthy habits, behaviors and thought patterns, will not go down easily. And no matter how successful he is, he will occasionally crave a drink. Whether he survives those times depends totally on how much of real "treatment" he has accepted and practices.

Sadly, most on-the-wagon over-drinkers will go ahead and get the drink—eventually. Just one, he tells himself. But that first drink of a "slip," a relapse, which doesn't get him drunk, does fire up the addiction again. It comes back fast, in full force—not starting all over at the beginning, but starting up back where he left off! His disorder is not like a cold or flu that get treated and then get well.

A sound way for you to think of "treatment" is always as merely "first-phase treatment." This first phase no more cures the problem than the first chemo treatment cures cancer.

In a nutshell: Do not bank on treatment as the solution.

* * *

If Not Treatment, Then What?

The combination of new knowledge and new techniques to deal with him and his behavior (remember that what he says, speaks, is also a behavior) will quickly begin changing your situation, almost always for the better. That doesn't mean he reforms; it means you either learn how to live "around" his situation, or learn how to separate. Though the tricks I'll show you are not at all difficult, they often don't come easily; they are sometimes scary, but always move you into a better position. The only exception is when the man has any tendency to violence. Then there are no known tricks that will straighten him out. That too is a sickness and it almost always only gets worse over time. Barring that, what you learn here will change your life. First it will change the way you think about what's going on, and second, it will give you new ways to respond to situations.

I'll show you why the approaches to changing him that others preach haven't worked (can't work), relieve your guilty feelings because you haven't forgiven or loved him "enough." Together, we'll fill your cart with new ways, tactics already proven to work for a drinker's woman. So by the time you finish this book you'll know quite well what's going on with him and understand it, *and* you'll have a boatload of new things to alter all of it.

In addition, we'll be taking a step back from the frustration and disappointment and hurt and chaos to examine what all that has been doing to you. And give you some solutions.

So who am I to be talking to you about all these things? I'm a licensed psychotherapist who has worked with drinkers's women and families for over 40 years. I also have the therapeutic advantage of having destroyed my own life by "over-drinking" and remember vividly how I thought and behaved (and have heard thousands over the years tell the same story). Further, I found solid, lasting recovery, sober and clean for over 44 years at this writing. And I remember all the things required by me and all other successes to do. Perhaps best of all, in terms of this book, during those lost and unhappy 20-plus years I lived with a nonspecific number of men who also drank too much (not with all of them at once, just one at a time). (Usually.) I really was just searching for love, not excitement, but excitement was what I got—if you understand that terror and anxiety are composed of the "excitement" brain chemicals. Anyway, most of the guys I chose (or who chose me) qualified for a full diagnosis of alcoholism. (Well, after all, who else would have me?)

Some of them had other problems too; chasing, gambling, not working, nose-picking, and (seriously) some were violent.

After years of struggling to achieve and maintain a sober mind, then become educated, certified, and licensed as a psychotherapist, I began applying some of the concepts born out of my own experience (and that of thousands of others I had by then become familiar with), to address issues in drinkers's families—especially in their women.

I've seen the huge change that occurs as women learn what is really going on with their guy, and why their attempts to change him never work (for long). They also quickly picked up a few simple tricks and—voila!—they overhauled their entire lives.

Women who picked up the simple ideas and tricks step by step report great life changes, the changes directly matched with how many old ways are toned down and how many new ways picked up.

As a result, I think I have something for you, for any woman who picks up this book, because its tricks often work as well on other people in their lives too.

Living with a man who drinks too much creates enough stress to begin to break his woman, whether he's a full alcoholic or not. Your interest in this of book tells me you're getting to the end of *your* rope. But here's some Good News: You're about to find many of the answers you've been looking for.

If you have suffered mental and emotional stress and pain associated with your mate's drinking, I want you to know that you have just stepped out on a short trip back to happy sanity.

I'm writing this book because I have learned things that haven't appeared in text books for psychology and counseling, thus not in the studies of people preparing to be counselors. And it's not found in other self-help books either. I'm writing this because I know the pain of a long-suffering woman, almost all of these are truly beautiful human beings, and the simple facts here have the power to change their lives. Readers have told me the book preceding this one already has, as well as a large number of women I worked with in therapy over the years.

Sadly, the messages in other books dealing with the over-drinker focus on telling you—the one who was originally okay, the one with the beautiful personality—what you should change. Trying to change yourself to fit the circumstances you now live with has already created the biggest part of your problems. You've been told to be more patient, kinder, more forgiving, more understanding, gentler, more loving—be better and do better, when you are already some of the most wonderful people on the planet. All this in order to deal with HIS problem. The over-all message is that your problem would be fixed if you change, do all the things they are urging on you.

The approach has been bought by "your kind of women." That's because your natural nature is to be generous, patient, loving, caring, good. It was easy to focus on those things you already do so well.

But it hasn't changed your situation for the better, has it?

I write this book because about 90 percent of women who are interested enough in its title and pick it up have been living in a gradually worsening life, like the poor frog put in the pot and the water gradually heated to boiling. You are beginning to stir and realize that your pot is getting too hot to sustain life.

Yet you have kept on keeping on, even as some of you have slid into desperation. Let's acknowledge that, for most of you, your pot is nearing the boiling point.

You have wondered why your guy has changed so much, why he started to blow up in anger, sometimes tiny things sparking huge rages; you've wondered why this man who used to tell you how wonderful you are, now stays on your back aid is so critical, unkind, seeming to be full of hatred. You wonder why he has quit being the sweet, cute, funny, romantic guy you fell in love with and become a—well, it's hard to name what he's become.

Perhaps the biggest reason I'm writing is because I've found that most of you hold the sense, perhaps a deep belief, that one day, one day, he's going to see the light! Then he'll straighten up and appreciate you and love you again.

This mistaken set of ideas was planted in you largely by your culture, our society, our movies, novels, TV shows, our music. Your dream of that great future includes his changing back into the great guy he was when you met and fell in love with him.

The Bad News: That will not happen for more than 90 percent of you who read this.

Millions of women have lived being mostly unhappy, and

they have aged far too soon from the stress, all because of these erroneous ideas. Who can blame all of us women for hanging onto the myths, they offer hope, and they are easier for you perhaps than for other women.

Most women of over-drinkers hang onto the myths of true love as strongly as the drinker hangs onto his ideas about finding euphoria, the feeling he is always seeking through drugging his brain with alcohol.

Having all these ideas to some degree, the drinker's woman who wants to help others, make them feel better, to please them, and that is not bad. And no, to regain your footing you don't stop trying to please others; you only make minor adjustments in how much you really want to give without getting what you need in return.

You now have a new ideal: Right now you are beginning to equal out pleasing yourself at least as often as you please others. And by realizing that not much in your life anymore actually depends on everybody loving you and thinking you're great. (When that idea, that you must please others, was formed you were only a crawling infant. Now, as a lovely and fully grown woman, you can look closer and see that your survival really does not depend on these people. You are capable of survival on your own should they all turn their backs on you. And, as you begin to toughen up, some of them probably will. These will be the ones who never really cared for you beyond what you could do or provide for them.

The infant's inner sense, belief, that her survival *did* depend on them was totally correct—but like many ideas formed in childhood, they don't hold when you grow up.

In this world, no matter how great you are, there will be people who will focus on your negatives. It is their ugly nature, their deformity. From this moment, however, you will see their misshapen souls as the problem, and not something about you. You will no longer let their deformed hearts influence the shape of your own.

As to the substance of your Belle and Beast, Snow White and Prince mindset, much research shows that it's extremely unlikely an over-drinker will get better at all.

Furthermore, even the handful who eventually move in that direction won't do it any time soon—which is an all-important idea for you. Take a step back from the action and assess how much longer you can (or want to) put up with things as they are—and rest assured that the over-drinker is going to get worse, not better. How much longer can you hold on without your own systems breaking down? More to the point, how much longer do you want to live the way you have been living, especially learning that the situation has only a tiny chance of getting better.

For some it seems strange that many women who have hung in there with an over-drinker who is one of the handful who actually does stop the downward slide, that she, after holding on so long through hell will file for divorce after he does better. For me that has never been a mystery: The dream is that he will be wonderful again, but he will not be. Cannot be. The true "alcoholic" will have drunk away the brain cells that house much of those personality qualities.

When the long-suffering wife-lover realizes that the dream is a bust, she finally lets go. She files for divorce.

In case you don't know, *any* drinker can quit drinking—for a while. But research shows that fewer than 10 percent can totally quit **and stay quit**. This means that even if something causes him to take a single step in the right direction, it has hardly any chance of doing any good for long.

How many times have women, and likely you, been crushed to see their guy who had been dry for a short while start nipping again. Or just stumble in drunk one evening.

Being able to quit (temporarily) does not mean that he has no problem with alcohol.

Countless women have been fooled by a drone time inker who frequently reminds them of how they stopped for three weeks or 11 months, you remember—back in 2001.

For some reason that in a bright light just doesn't make sense, most people believe that if a person can stop at all, he doesn't have a problem. This is not so! Here's what tells you inescapably that he has a drinking problem:

He has a drinking problem if his drinking causes problems, any kind of problems.

Once contracted, the basic "sickness" doesn't ever go away; he will never return to drinking without eventually being sucked back down to his lowest level—most likely sooner than later.

Proof that he doesn't have a problem isn't that he can quit; he proves that he *does* have a problem when he doesn't stay quit.

The brain changes from the corrosive effect of alcohol are damages that will *not* get well, will not grow back. As with stroke victims and others with brain damage, sometimes they can learn how to do something all over again, but often, they cannot—at last at the level they expect.

All of this is to help you see more clearly that for you to hold on, hang in, in the face of actual abuse, mental and emotional even if not physical.

It is likely that you have been struggling to tolerate the intolerable based on your Inner Child's belief in fairy tale endings—specifically, that at some point, always down the road, he's going to, if *only* you hang in and do right, see the light and make a huge change—become your prince again (even a decent man) and you will live happily ever after. Fairy tales.

One of the greatest human fears is of the unknown, and the future is unknown; therefore, it's natural that much anxiety attaches to risky life decisions. It would be no surprise to find that his critical judgements of you over time have chipped away your confidence, the sheer repetition of his negative thoughts about you giving rise to the idea that you can't make it on your own, or in any way without depending on him.

It brings quick relief from anxiety to just discard thoughts of your unknown future if you change anything fundamental—such as your partner or residence. That brief sense of relief is so sweet as to encourage to drop that idea, or believe it's impossible for you. Occurring time after time, negative experiences associated in any way with his drinking can grind you down, and crash you if you count on his latest vow to stop drinking. The terrible letdown, often emergencies because he didn't take care of business or whatever when he was depended on. Grinding your life away, your hope away, your faith in the future.

The dream that somewhere down the road, the fairy tale that he will change, the fantasy of the two of you living happily ever after is not only false, which hurts to contemplate, but worse: Believing it sets you up to be hurt even worse. Part of what you will do here is begin to understand exactly why your dream cannot come true.

I hope I've burst your bubble. And I assure that all this Bad News will soon seem to turn into Good News.

Getting Specific

Psychological research has revealed that just wanting change will never work. For you to accomplish real change, you first must get a clear picture of exactly what you want (to the best of your ability at this time).

Try this: Imagine that you have a wonderful, sparkling magic wand and you can wave over your guy and he will –well, what? What would you want to happen?

_____

Getting clear on the answer to that question is the beginning of real change. What exactly do you want to come about?

If you answer, "He'd be my prince again," there's a chapter here on that. If you answer, "He would be gone!" there's a chapter on that too!

Next, let's look at the some of the things you've already tried to get him to change (things we know didn't work because he didn't change, or didn't stay changed or you wouldn't be reading this book). We look at things you've already tried because it's important for you to absorb the fact that they don't work. Why do you need to do that? To save you time and trouble, and add years to your life. To improve your potato-rosemary soup.

List some of the things you've already tried to get him to straighten up. (Don't forget "scream, cuss, cry, and threatening to leave," "throw things, get drunk yourself, run away, come back, run away, come back, run away . . . .)

1. _____

2. _____

3. _____

4. _____

5. _____

(Put any other tactics you think of on Note Pages in the back of this book or a notebook journal. Ideally, over the next two or three weeks, you'll remember others.) You'll benefit from keeping track of things you've tried already without much success. Keeping track makes it easier to stop yourself when you start the same-old with him.

The next step is to start watching for the human tendency to repeat these things you've already tried that haven't worked.

For some, circling those items will cause it to imprint on the subconscious more firmly, thus helping you catch yourself when responding to him out of reflex starts. (And you will, many times.)

So what have you tried? Talking to him? Fussing at him? Threatening to leave? Crying? Pitching a fit? Getting drunk yourself? Leaving (then coming back)? Trying but failing to stay silent when goaded? Honestly speaking your mind?

And did any of those work? Cause him to change?

Taking a minute to picture doing each of these things gives you additional strength—it strengthens your subconscious sense of what you want to watch for. This alone for some is sufficient to begin halting repeating them again and again, always expecting that they just might work this time (even though you always see later that they didn't).

A note on picking up new techniques: No matter if a self-control trick worked for someone else, when you find it doesn't work for you after a few tries, it's time to move on. Look for and practice another trick with the promise of getting you desired results, always remembering that it's not a deficit in you if a trick doesn't come easily or work as well as you wish. All of us differ in every tiniest part of our personalities and abilities, and it is just fine for you to be okay with yourself just as the Manufacturer made you. Those differences aren't problems, but helps for you to do all the good things that were intended for you when you were shaped. Finding new tricks once you've run through all those in this book is simple; you almost always find what you need in self-help books in the library or book store. Get books on CDs free from your public library and listen to them as you run about in your car. You'll be amazed how much you can pick up this way.

If something you tried in the past seemed to work, but soon he fell back into the same old same old, then you must face the fact that it actually did not work.

We're not looking for something to make him nice for a few days or weeks, and then slip back to the same old stuff. We discard the methods that don't work. When you fix a leaky faucet and it gradually gets back as bad in a few days or weeks, you don't consider that your fix worked. Dump that fix for *that* problem. (Many fixes, however, won't work on one situation, yet do fine in another.)

Listing the things you've already tried to get him to change has the effect of helping you "catch it" when using one of them again comes to mind.

An extremely distressing error lies behind your mindset, your idea, belief, that something you can do or say to stop him from doing something, or start doing something can possibly work without the use of deadly force.

And especially is there nothing you've ever tried that stopped him and then caused him to stay stopped.

Staying aware that tactics you've used in the past haven't worked will save you much disappointment and stress, and it can add years to your life (which years will be far happier than otherwise).

* * *

For over 40 years I've been meeting, getting to know, and coming to love hundreds of women who likely have been so much like you. What I've learned from these hundreds of women is that they turn out to be surprisingly similar. *All* of them have the truest, gentlest, and kindest form of loving and giving. They have suffered for the benefit of others, especially the drinker, often for their children they have endured the unendurable, sometimes paying a very high cost.

No other kind of woman would have lived in or put up with what you have.

A woman in a relationship with a man who drinks too much is always a giver. Others would have given up long ago. She'll be compassionate, and we know that because otherwise she would have booted him after the first or second mess-up. She'll love hard, and she'll deeply care about others (although, some of you may be running low in that particular quality at the moment; nevertheless, it is one of your strong personality traits). This woman will have more than average patience, especially with those she loves (which also is likely running short about now), and she also tends to forgive, and *forget* all but the most damaging mistreatments. Indeed, the women we are talking about are some of the most precious souls on earth. They are made to love—and to be loved. To be all those things takes a heck of a woman. (They find these facts particularly hard to accept. Why do you suppose that is? Much of it is, once again, traits and ways of thinking dating from childhood—and that's Good News because it means they can be adjusted to more realistic levels.

You've already proved all of these really good things about yourself by just picking up this book. You have to be one of those types of women to be here.

If you are in a relationship that feels like a trap—it would have required possessing all of the traits we've just covered, and more, for you to have been able to stick with him this long. This is who you really are.

But you're with a guy who has assuredly harmed you at least emotionally and mentally, if not physically. You care about a man who has been turning your life upside down. What kind of woman would stay? Right: Great love, strength, generosity, forgiving. Not because you're stupid, which you likely have accused yourself of being, but it's because you are the special kind of person we've been talking about. Take a breath here and picture yourself wearing all those traits.

It doesn't take a crystal ball to see that anyone other than a giving, forgiving, compassionate, caring, and strong woman would have kicked his sorry--uh,—wouldn't have stayed long enough to get to the point where you are now.

I also found out something else about the woman who lives with a man who drinks too much: Get this: She's spunky!

Yeah. You may think that spunky part of you has been driven underground, or laid down and pulled the covers over her head, but you are wrong. Indeed, it's the spunky part of you that picked up this book. It's that part of you that has stayed, because she's not stopping looking for still other ways to set him right—and her own life right.

Your spunk has been twisted a bit (maybe kicked around and stomped on) but the proof that it's still alive and well is that you're still here fighting the problem, looking for solutions to a situation that has gotten pretty bad. That takes spunk, girl.

As long as you can stomp your foot, throw a glass, call him a bad name, and make up your mind to do something about your situation, you've still got more spunk than the average gal. Or guy, for that matter. In fact, it's your natural spunk that I'm betting on to revive your spirit and stoke your fire, to fire you up with the ideas you'll be getting here.

Every thing you've tried in the past to fix your relationship has been hatched in a very good mind. Your kind of good mind is always on the lookout for more ideas to try out (witness your reading this book). We look at this because it's still more of the incredible personality package that is you. All of these things are not stupid, as he may sometimes label you. (You'll learn why: For starters, he has to do it to convince himself that whatever you say about his behavior is worthless.)

You've been using your high quality (over-worked and over-stressed) mind to survive, but your problems arise because you don't fully understand what you are up against; hence, your attempts have failed. (To you failure may have meant you were inadequate, but the truth is that your tactics and what you aim at are what have failed you. You've been firing your great shots in the dark, not understanding your true target. The trap that has snared you is that sometimes your attempts seem to succeed. But then they fall apart—again. And you feel worse then than you did before you tried to fix things.)

Those failures have led you to doubt yourself, but again, you aren't what's failing; it's the tactics and targets doing that. My heart breaks knowing almost all of you condemn yourselves for those failures. You may sometimes even question your sanity.

The answer comes by stepping back and analyzing the situation. It's abnormal. Have you recognized that so far?

It's abnormal because you don't have the usual kind of relationship problems—well, you do but they are all twisted up and made worse with extras that others don't usually have.

Here's a new mindset to work with: You have, up to now, been relying on tools and tactics made for normal people in normal situations.

Most of them are just fine—*for normal problems, but most normal* responses won't work with someone who is drinking too much. *This is because they and the situations they create are abnormal—out of the ordinary. Those tactics just take up space in your playbook.*

Think of your old tactics like a football team diving into the game with tennis rackets. Or firemen trying to put out a fire with donuts. You just haven't been equipped with the tools needed for your specific jobs. Your failures are not because you are lacking, because you are not. They are due to a lack of information.

When your temper blows, I'll guarantee you that whatever the last straw was is far beyond where most others would have held on. So you can drop thinking that you're weak. Weakness is not your problem. We now are going to change out your equipment, give you a new tool box, in fact, you'll be getting an entire new bag of tricks.

When you start thinking that you're going crazy, it's because you find yourself doing things not common for you—or doing something someone else says is bad or crazy. (Soon we'll examine exactly who says these things to you—and how you can change the power they wield.) Others often self-boosting judgements of you have created much of your self-doubt. If others treated you as if you were below par, below the norm, or they withheld their approval or love because of your failure to meet some demand, those are the things that create a harsh inner critic. The process is the same whether you're an infant or a grown woman.

Temper fits or crying jags, you know, are perfectly normal—especially for a woman who lives in an abnormal situation, with a man who drinks too much. When one faces a changeable personality, with cruelty in their speech and actions, when one has her nest rattled, shaken, shredded, and with it her security and dreams, it is perfectly normal to pitch a fit.

But you felt like you'd done something wrong. Likely others condemned your anger too. Now ask yourself, What kind of woman would sit quietly by when her nest was being shaken apart, when she saw her dreams being busted up, her whole life ripped apart by another's thoughtless (and abnormal) behavior?

While there are millions of women in this country in situations almost identical to yours, that doesn't make the conditions you live with "normal." They are quite abnormal. Your reactions turn out to be perfectly normal for anyone facing the same things.

So you are not crazy, and you are spunky. For now, take my word for it.

Until now, most books written to women about their men's drinking aim at salvaging the drinker. And they urge his woman to get him into some form of treatment—like that's now her job. Like that's going to work. It's no coincidence that many of these books are written by people who work for big treatment centers.

That focus is not what you'll find here, mainly because it rarely works. And when it does, it has a high rate of falling back.

No, this book focuses not so much on salvaging him but on salvaging you.

Together we will accomplish that by laying out little-known, often deliberately hidden, information, by explaining some of the troublesome changes you've seen in him so you can better counter them, and by showing you multiple ways to more successfully interact with him and cut off some of his nastiest trees at their roots. What you probably don't know now about what's really going on with him can be the death of you. Literally.

You'll be learning some new "tricks" here, each one guaranteed to give you more control over your relationship and yourself, and find out that most can actually be fun. Actually, these will be tactics, techniques—but it sounds like more fun when we call them "tricks." And many of them are great fun.

We're going to talk about men who drink too much here; I refer to them as "over-drinkers," so let's clarify that now: "Over-drinking" doesn't necessarily mean alcoholic, so using "over-drinker" bypasses some sticky issues. "Over-drinking" is simply drinking too much.

And how much is too much? It's drinking enough that it interferes with his life. And yours. To the point where it changes his personality, where he develops new behavior—bad behavior. All of this happens, yet he doesn't give up the drinking! (Well, he may occasionally give it up, but he just can't make that last.)

In other words: He can quit. He just can't stay quit. As a mental health professional, I tell you that anyone who continues doing something harmful to himself, or things and people he cares about, isn't normal. Not only is it not normal, it is not sane. The strongest instinct in humans (and animals) is the survival instinct; consequently, continued self-harming behavior flies in the face of the supposedly number one, overwhelming drive to survive. And makes his behavior seriously abnormal. Which makes the person doing it seriously abnormal. Doing things that go against one's survival instinct is used as grounds for commitment.

You, my darling girl, are an incredibly beautiful personality type; he, in contrast, is becoming seriously abnormal. But he's the one who keeps suggesting that you're the one who is abnormal!

Okay: My message in the bottle is this: It's him—not you.

* * *

Preview of What's Coming

- You are going to find that his drinking is at the bottom of far more of your relationship problems than you thought.
- You'll see how his behavior when drinking too much creates stress on you that seriously affects your emotional, mental, and physical health.
- The emotional damage an over-drinker inflicts on his woman with his behavior and his words can stay with her for life—unless addressed in very specific ways (meaning she gets knowledgeable help, and she is not treated as having simple anxiety or depression).
- You'll begin to see and understand that he's not likely to get better—and stay that way—and why.
- You'll understand why, if he continues to drink any alcohol at all, he'll only get worse. (This is guaranteed. That's because most of his negative changes are due to very real damage alcohol is doing to his brain cells.)
- You'll understand that many of the signs professionals are currently required to use to diagnose and pronounce that someone has a drinking problem don't even show up until a drinker is almost beyond recall, totally due to the extent of that brain damage. He won't have the brain strength needed to make the difficult changes required.
- You'll get a diagnostic chart that lets you diagnose his drinking problem for yourself.
- You'll learn techniques to more successfully interact with him—drunk or sober.
- You'll learn techniques to avoid or escape arguments.
- You'll learn techniques to prevent being hurt by the mean things he says.
- You'll learn techniques for taking back control of how your own life flows.
- You'll learn techniques for making your life better, much better—no matter what he chooses to do with his life.
- You'll learn how to make a decision about what's best for you—To Go? To Stay? To Send Him Away?

- Oh yes—you'll also begin learning how you may have become a setup for bad relationships in the first place. Best of all, we'll sneak a peek at what you can do about that.

* * *

What You've Been Dealing With

His problem, sadly, is due to in large part to things he has had his genetic makeup, no control over: his genetics and other heredity, and the way he learned to cope with life. While it's sad, no one can be expected to live with someone actively destroying everything around him.

We avoid the word "alcoholic." It's a label; it's misleading. It seems to blame the substance alcohol when, in fact, problem drinking is due solely to things inside the drinker. Proof of that is that we don't have any "rat-poison-aholics." In the 1930s, our society accepted a new name for an ancient disorder; it was a name invented to lessen the shame of having a drinking problem, a name that cut down the use of demeaning words such as a drunk, a sot, and worse.

The new word also made it easier for the imbiber to seek help; that new name was "alcoholism." This name change worked for 70 or 80 years, but now that new name, "alcoholic," has become the new demeaning label, distasteful, especially to the drinker, as the old-fashioned terms. You may have noticed that those with the disorder react strongly to the word "alcoholic" (perhaps more strongly than the old-timers did to "drunkard," and "sot.")

But all that's changed is the name: Over-drinkers's behavior didn't change because it had a new name. It is apparent that an over-drinker by any other name still smells as bad.

And they all drink for the same reason: It changes the way they feel. Such a simple concept driving such a devastating life choices.

Your Foundational Trick

Start now eliminating (best you can) the word "alcoholic" from all conversation with him. The word is a fire-starter, a short fuse on a bomb. Over-drinkers go bananas when you use the words "alcoholic" and "alcoholism" in any way associated with them. Only use the word "alcoholic" when you're ready to set fire to the house.

The mental picture of what a "drunk," or "alcoholic" is continues in the public mind as someone homeless and rag-tag. This stereotype, however, turns out to be a picture of many real "alcoholics" or over-drinkers, but only in the last stage. Most people judge the seriousness of a drinking problem by comparing the over-drinker they see to the stereotype. (That picture, by the way, is one of a man too late to save.)

Our culture continues to hold the idea that drinking isn't really a problem until it gets to "that" level—meaning the level of the stereotype "drunk." This terribly mistaken idea remains deeply rooted in our cultural mind, despite reams of evidence that a drinker's disintegration and entrapment is real long, long before he gets that bad. It's like refusing to call it "cancer" until the tumor is eight inches across.

Another victim of social stereotype is the drinker's woman. The impact of his escalating disorder on her also starts long, long before he gets "that bad."

It's usually his woman who first sees that he has a problem. She also will see most of the worst of it. All the while, the rest of the world may call him a jackass, but not an "alcoholic." As for his woman, the rest of the world has been known to say that he's the way he is because she's such a nag, or coo-coo.

For some drinkers, the bad behavior begins as soon as their drinking does. For others, it begins shortly after, and for others— not until long after. No one considers or accepts that the bad behavior brought onto her, forced on her, is what causes a drinker's woman's terrible decline. To confuse things further, there is no true definition of the word "alcoholism." The best definition we have is just the list of signs professionals use to diagnose it. It's like saying a cold is only sniffles and coughs and a sore throat, rather than explaining the precise cause of those signs. The signs currently used to diagnose drinking problems are like diagnosing heart trouble as "a heart attack," or cancer diagnosed by "sickness and death." In other words, current diagnosing of an over-drinker diagnoses by Last Stage damage the alcohol has done. Most who survive to reach Last Stage will not be able to make it back—due to the damage sustained.

Another thing is that labels like "alcoholic" or "drunk" don't take into account what a drinker was like before he became such a mess. But you do. (And that tendency, holding on to the image of what he used to be, has cost you, and millions upon millions of other women, a large chunk of your and their lives.)

Even though you've watched him change into what he's become, your original idea of who he was still colors who you think he is today. (Not coincidentally, what he used to be is largely what has held you with him, even though other women would have been long gone—it's that image of who and what he once was.) It's no longer real. It's like being in love with a fantasy.

The problem is that you tend to believe he's still that. Remembering how sweet he used to be, longing for that to come back, and believing it can be done, if only . . . you add, if only . . . fill in the blank. That idea is part of the deadly trap that holds you.

Likely, before you came looking for this book, your drinker was already at the Middle Stages of his disintegration (when their personalities are changing noticeably, and their behaviors are becoming alarming). But one part of you still tends to think of him as the man he was before he got this bad, and it's coupled with the belief that something you do or say will make him go back to being that other man. This thinking has held your feet to the fire as it burns ever hotter.

An over-drinker by any other name still smells (and behaves) as bad.

Fact: Your belief that he can and will go back to Prince, as well as that this can happen due to something you do or say—that's the dream. It's the fantasy in the old stories you read as a child (perhaps still being reinforced by stories you read now). Both those beliefs are erroneous. He isn't and will never again be the guy you fell in love with. Some few do "recover," which means they stop drinking. Even fewer will be sweeter. But the lost brain parts will not grow back.

By Middle Stage and beyond, nothing you an say or do will fix him. If someone is lying about his drinking, sneaking drinks, drinking until he passes out, slurring words after starting to drink, his hands trembling, increasingly withdrawing from you and his home life, less and less caring about and tending to elements of his life separate from drinking, and denying he has a problem—well, that's danged serious.

Professional diagnoses only give a name to signs that have been there all along; they're just getting more serious. The same problem that kept getting worse—the little lump that kept getting bigger, the occasional arrhythmia that kept getting worse.

The problem with current professional guidelines for diagnosing whether someone is in trouble with drinking is that when they are finally allowed (by guidelines of their licenses) to diagnose them as needing help, more than 90 percent of the time, it's too late.

Only a handful of over-drinkers reaching that point, the point where they manifest the signs currently required to get them meaningful help, will ever get free and stay that way.

For a diagnosing professional to see the deterioration currently required for diagnosis and treatment (and for insurance to help pay for it) profound changes in the body and brain of he drinker must already have occurred. Most of those signs arise from body and brain deterioration.

That much deterioration robs the brain of the mental ability required to get free—and stay that way. (The brain cells required to "just say no" are gone. The brain cells controlling behavior, whether he reaches for a drink or not, and his judgement, are all damaged).

To make our current approach still less effective, most assessments of a drinking problem are conducted solely by talking to the drinker! Of all the people in the world to correctly judge and diagnose a drinking problem, the worst person is someone whose brain is not only terribly damaged but who also has a strong need to continue getting the feelings alcohol gives. Professionals ask the drinker questions that a fool could see will get him in trouble if he answers honestly—so he won't.

Sometimes he doesn't even realize he's lying—or doesn't realize how seriously he's lying. He may realize he's shading the truth, but hides from himself how profound his untruths are. That warped information continues to be the primary diagnostic tool. Even so, what he admits is often more than enough to show serious change as well as brain damage. But those easy-to-see signs of trouble currently aren't considered enough to rate intervention.

The behavior of an over-drinker is the only reliable key to diagnosis, and that must be from the point of view of several other people close to him. Obtaining these outside observations, and then interviewing the drinker, the diagnosing therapist can use those observations of others close to him to refute his half-truths and downright lies. This form of confrontation appears to be the most potent game-changer for over-drinkers. This is the value of friend-and-family led interventions.

But understand—all of that is not enough to get him sober and keep him sober. All it can do it allow him to see that he needs help, become open for effective treatment. The over-drinker won't let on to the truth until it's way too late for treatment to be able to help him. By the time the brain parts that hold what we call "denial" are also damaged (eaten away) enough for the truth to pop out, so is the rest of his brain. Including those parts needed to get out and especially, to stay out.

To repeat: The worst person in the world from whom to get accurate information about a drinker's drinking is the drinker! The best is the woman who lives with him.

* * *

You Can Better Understand His Behavior By Understanding What's Happening to His Body

Alcohol (a toxic, depressant drug) is an anesthetic. It kills the experience of pain by affecting brain cells. Problem is that it takes very little alcohol to damage a brain cell, and when a brain cell is damaged, even slightly, it starts failing, and begins to die.

Within seconds the cell's function is impaired. That means his behavior can also change that fast. Brain cell damage and death follows even slight damage to the cell. This means the area of brain where that cell was located is now vacant—permanently useless. It won't grow back. If the cell is in the judgement center, the drinker's judgement is rapidly affected. In seconds.

Alcohol dulls brain cells, like morphine and heroin (also invented as anesthetics). Working on body cells with an acidic effect, alcohol abrades and weakens cell walls, pulls out their fluid, leaving the cell's little inner parts drying and dying. While slightly tougher, other body cells are still delicate; alcohol affects them the same way. The major difference: They usually can grow back, except liver cells.

Cells of the liver, kidney, digestive system, skin, lungs, cardio system, and all the rest are exposed to the acidic effect of alcohol. They too are affected and impaired. It's just that other organs, as they are losing their functions, don't affect his behavior in the total way brain cells do. Loss of a liver cell, even a liver patch, doesn't turn him into a horse's butt. A disintegrating liver doesn't make him think he's just fine and everybody else is nuts, doesn't make him spend money foolishly or treat his woman badly.

Body cells are delicate little packages, skins, sacs, holding fluid. Floating in that fluid are incredibly tiny little parts (called organelles). They float around, busy doing the work of the particular cell, for example, producing digestive juices or infection fighters or sweat or urine. And brain cells are the one of the first hit body cells by alcohol in the blood.

Just as an abrasion, like a skinned knee, can cause body cells to spring a leak, so does alcohol affect body cells. The little working parts inside a cell can't make their way around to do their jobs if they spring a leak and begin to dry out. Now they can't get the nourishment they need, they can't eliminate the waste they create. That cell loses its ability to function, and then it dies—usually by poisoning itself with its own waste. This is the same process we see when our bodies sprung a leak: Our organs could no longer do their work; they require lots of clean water and nourishment. Our organs can't take in nourishment or rid themselves of their natural waste. The body holding these organs would die. (This way of working on the human body explains why the legal drug alcohol is correctly classified as "toxic.")

Alcohol enters the bloodstream within seconds of hitting the lips. It isn't necessary to swallow and digest alcohol for it to get into the blood and also be sent to the cells of the body; it's absorbed before swallowing by the tissues of the mouth, tongue, and the entire "tube" of the digestive system. Around 20 percent of the alcohol is already absorbed into the blood before the rest of that swallow reaches his stomach. It's already hitting the brain. Upon entering the bloodstream, it is carried by the blood (which races around the body at high speed, 60 to 90 heart pumps per minute), touching every single living cell in the body on every single pass. Round and round and round it goes. Touching cells, gradually abrading, damaging and killing.

(Note: A drinker's behavior, early in a bout, doesn't look like he's taking poison. He seems happy—carefree—which, by the by is the feeling that drives him to drink! It's not that you burned the steak or weren't nice to him. But most of the good feelings a drinker gets is simply the result of brain cells being put out of order. When muscles relax, it's because their cells are abraded and weakened; it's not a good thing.)

Alcohol slams the cells of liver and kidneys, those organs

whose major job is to rid the body of toxins! That means, as they try to do their jobs, their cells slug down and die, are damaged and then destroyed. Their function weakens with every hit as the alcohol comes back in the blood continuously until broken down. They become so damaged these organs no longer work. Fewer healthy cells on each alcohol pass through the kidney and liver means that less alcohol can be broken down, and that means the alcohol just stays in the blood longer and longer, continuing to hit every body cell over and over. Round and round.

How His Deterioration and Debilitation Affect You

A drinker's woman is affected from the very start; she also sees what others don't, all but his most hidden acts—and she usually suspects even those. While she may be afraid or ashamed to tell anyone what she knows, she holds more of the truth than will be found anywhere else. An accredited therapist will be able to help her open up.

Accurate and useful diagnosis of a drinking problem is currently confused by the common belief (sometimes held even by professionals) that the drinker's past is "the reason" he over-drinks. Most people judge the problem less harshly if there is some terrible life experience that they believe is at the bottom of it.

It's true that for many drinkers that a life trauma can spur them into a increased use, to dull the terrible mental and emotional discomfort left by the event. This increased drinking, if it lasts eve for months is almost guaranteed to create enough brain changes to intensify the drinking still more. Once he begins drinking enough for the damage to begin at a higher rate, no matter how or why it started, he is in trouble.

This is why you can't excuse either his drinking or his bad behavior out of sympathy. In almost every case, the groundwork for developing a drinking problem was already there—in his genetics and the way he learned to cope with life—here long before the trauma hit and he chose the path of dulling his feelings with the toxic, depressant drug alcohol.

But he never knew how bad that could turn out.

What can we do to be sure young people today know?

(Note: Research shows that the younger a man was when he began drinking, the less likely is he to recover. This is true irrespective of any trauma experience. An over-drinker will

glom onto and expand an everyday bad experience until it seems to justify his desire to drink. If you need proof of this, note that there are multiple millions of people walking around today who have experienced as bad an experience as he has just used as an excuse—and worse—but they don't over-drink because of it.)

VERY IMPORTANT

Information to Know Up-Front
(Otherwise, he'll fool you because he probably doesn't know these things himself. When he says, "It was just a few beers," now you know something he doesn't!)

Amount of alcohol in a regular mixed drink:
1½ ounces of alcohol

Amount of alcohol in a five-ounce glass of wine:
1½ ounces of alcohol

Amount of alcohol in an 8-ounce can of beer
1½ ounces of alcohol

The healthy body breaks down alcohol at the rate of about ¾-ounce an hour. The above chart means it will take approximately two hours to remove the bulk of the alcohol from just *one* drink.

(Note: A great misconception many people still hold is that if a person is not drinking at the moment, or if he has had only one or two drinks, there's no problem with him driving—especially if it's "**only**" wine or beer he's been drinking, which, as you just saw, are wrongly considered lesser villains.)

Many drinkers's women believe that what a man drinks or how much he drinks is the measure of his problem. But, as you've just seen, it isn't particularly important what form of alcohol a man drinks—beer, wine, or whiskey—the outcome is the same. Now you understand why. Whatever he's drinking, by the time it is interfering so much that his woman calls it a problem—he's already hooked, caught. The toxin has done a mass of damage, especially to his brain cells, and that's why. The substance that does the damage is present in the same amount in all of those drinks.

Drinking "hard liquor" only makes "the feeling" come on faster. The alcohol it contains is exactly the same substance that is in wine and beer.

As to how much he drinks, remember that the true amount he drinks is always a guessing game. If you think he's drinking too much, judging by what you know, it is certain he's already drinking a good bit that you don't know about. Even he doesn't know for sure—but you can bet won't admit all that he does know.

Why is this? Because a part of him knows that those things would "suggest" that he has a problem, and he will do anything to avoid people saying that. Why? Because he knows they would demand that he stop drinking. And getting "that feeling" has become too important, and while becoming insane, he's not stupid. He lies about it. Sometimes even to himself.

When he doesn't lie about the amount, he lies to himself about its effect on him.

The *amount* of whatever he drinks is a factor in the speed of his deterioration, the speed of personality change , the breakdown of his body—but again, you have no way of knowing just how much he's *really* been consuming. How much he drinks is only one of many signs that give the unquestionable diagnosis of his problem.

Things not so easily observed as what he actually drinks have more to do with becoming an over-drinker. A man's genetic inheritance (some of his organs may be just a little short of tiny cells needed for processing alcohol, or such); his over-all health is a large part of it (for a similar reason); his body size, because it has to do with how much alcohol is in his blood. (A 200-pound man would have less alcohol-to-blood than 150=pound man because his he has less blood to dilute it); how he learned to handle the twists of life—how flexible are his skills at dealing with stress. All of these things determine his tipping point. Of course, all those things are made worse, weaker, with every drink.

But what marks a man as an over-drinker is his behavior—his behavior before, during, and after drinking.

If his behavior and-or his personality change for the worse once he starts drinking, that is sufficient sign to diagnose that he is already in trouble, and on a deadly path. The reasoning goes back to the survival instinct rule. You can take a shortcut here by looking at whether, when he quits, he can stay quit.

What's more, when his drinking begins interfering with his life (and yours), you don't need a professional to tell you he has a serious drinking problem. He does. We know that because the survival instinct is wired to get rid of anything that isn't good for us. But his isn't working, despite the toxicity and destructive life effects.

His drinking of the toxic depressant drug alcohol isn't what's most important to you. What's important to you is what his drinking does (and has been doing) to him, to his body, his mind, and the behavior it is producing in him.

Soon we'll take a look at what all of that is doing to you.

What Drives Him?

The definition of "sanity" is based in largest measure on a person's instinct for survival. Thus, when drinking begins to slam around any important segment of his life, a sane person quits. Sane people quit doing things that harm them. All it takes in most states to have you committed is to show that you have lost the will or ability to keep yourself from harm. Something has gone seriously wrong in the man who becomes an over-drinker.

Making it more confusing, the over-drinker relies totally on the "good" feelings that alcohol produces in him as proof that it's not bad. He uses the impressions from a drugged and damaged brain to assess himself! And those very "good feelings" are the sole reason an over-drinker over-drinks. He wants to get them again. worse, the "good feelings" are simply the effect he gets from his drug of choice, an effect he sees as relief. (For Pete's sake, distilled spirits were invented as an anesthetic for removing limbs on the battleground! Yer durn tootin' it brings relief.) The alcohol (a toxic depressant drug) has affected the nerve cells that are his brain. First and most seriously affected? His judgement.

You know—the part of his brain that judges when he's had enough, or it's time to stop, or go home.

Once any behavior begins to negatively affect one's life, a healthy, sane person with sound judgement stops that behavior.

If he doesn't stop, that in itself is a sign of what can be a serious mental health disorder. Indeed, that very thing is the primary reason people are forcibly put into mental health treatment—they don't stop doing something harmful to themselves (or others).

Continuing a self-harming behavior is considered insanity when the harm is serious. We can say that because survival is the strongest set of instincts in most living creatures, especially humans. Yet the over-drinker casts those instincts aside—the effects on his job, health, finances, family life, and those around him—as well as his own increasing misery.

Then they get all crossed up; he begins to follow the crazy ways in the deep belief they are his only way to survival. His survival mechanism has been fatally twisted. His drinking, his playing, his spending. His drinking and the behavior it produces can be sufficient signs of serious mental disorder. In short, he's not quite sane at best.

And with this understanding is how you will, from this very moment, interpret everything he does, and especially everything he says to you. Sometimes it may come from his residual sanity, but you never know which thing he's saying comes from there. This reminds me of an ancient story about two sages, one who always speaks the truth, and the other one always lies. The problem here is like yours: No one knows which one is speaking, the one who speaks truth or the one who lies.

The ancient solution: Don't rely on what either one says!

Over-drinkers have an early phase of their drinking when it doesn't appear to do them much damage. As well, in the beginning the type of drinks, the frequency of drinking, and the amounts consumed can differ widely among drinkers. But that's only in the beginning. As the drink affects his brain, his behavior unravels due to changes in his brain, and those changes are the same in all brains being assailed by over-drinking. The result: He will gradually become more and more like all other over-drinkers. He cannot escape a bitter end. No one stays a happy drunk for long.

One of the first changes I want you to make is switching your focus off of his drinking and onto how the things he does affect you. How does his behavior (words and actions) affect you?

_____Do you get tense, just thinking about him starting to drink?
_____Do you fear for his safety? Spend time with worry-anxiety chemicals flooding your body?
_____Do you fear for your safety?
_____Do you fear for your family's safety when he's been drinking and demands the right to drive?
_____Are you distressed (anxiety), angry, losing sleep, distracted and out of focus during the day, anxious, depressed, and worse?
_____Are you emotionally distraught?
_____Are you frequently stressed?
_____Are you lonely?

* * *

I Remember . . . Only Having Two Beers
A few years before I fell out of love with destroying myself, I learned that I could have my cake and eat it too. I was beginning to be embarrassed when anyone asked me how much I drank. About that time, I began drinking my beer by the quart, my liquor in bigger glasses; then I could say I only had one or two beers, one or two drinks--and I wouldn't be lying.
(I'm not the only one who has figured out this scam!)

* * *

More About Effects of Alcohol on Body Cells
Alcohol damages body cells. Over-drinking it destroys them.
More to the point, drinking more in a twenty-four hour period than a given body can process (the body's ability to chemically break down and get the toxic drug alcohol out of the body) means the mass of alcohol is left circulating in his blood, touching every cell in his body, doing its damage, over and over as his heart pumps the alcohol-laden blood around and around and through his body.
If one drinks additional alcohol before his body has time to repair (best it can) the last damages, the new influx of alcohol adds its effects to the old that's still there—and if it's there, it's

active. Picture the body working hard to break down a toxin, any poison, and get it out of the system, working at the peak of its strength--while the same body pours in still more alcohol. What's happening is like pouring more poison in while the body is desperately trying to destroy the last dose.

Not giving the body the time it needs to repair injury before adding new toxin is how alcohol damage rapidly accumulates. The healthy body breaks down and ejects alcohol at the rate of about ¾-ounce per hour. That means the most healthy body takes at least two full hours to clear the alcohol from one drink from the liver and kidney and blood—of just one drink.

Unfortunately, the cells alcohol damages first and most are in his brain and the organs needed to break down and excrete alcohol! The brain—which we expect to tell him when he's had enough--after one drink, it's affected—brain cells are closing down, his judgement is instantly affected. He cannot fully realize how he is being changed, not sufficiently to decide to stop it. After just one drink (one beer!), the brain centers that are supposed to tell him he's had enough are already out of kilter.

All of this explains how the changes in your man's personality are the direct result of alcohol's toxic effect on his body cells— more specifically, his brain cells. Indeed, most of you can see differences in his behavior and personality after just one drink.

I remember a film back in college of examining the brains of deceased alcoholics. What you see is the brain mass gouged with great empty holes, huge gaps in the usual spongy tissue. Those gaps are why, after a certain point, he can never again be the man you fell in love with again. Those brain cells, their skills and memories, are dead. They do not grow back. indeed, much of those gaps are where his judgement and control once resided. Gone now.

In order to halt the brain's deluded drive to self-destruction, we professionals must begin diagnosing sooner—much sooner. In Chapter 5 I've given a more thorough list of observable signs of a serious drinking problem. This expanded diagnostic guide will help you make your own diagnosis of his drinking and use that to help you make decisions. You don't have to wait for him to go to some professional (even his doctor) and be completely honest about his drinking. (Which won't happen until the very, very end, if he lives that long. Even then, he'll shade it.)

Undoubtedly, the most serious consequences of over-drinking actually land on the drinker's woman. His condition gets lots of press, but it's damaging many of you as much or more than him.

What Are You Looking For Here?

Let's tune your brain settings to get the greatest benefit from what you read here. Get specific about what you're looking for in this book, what you really want to find out and list them below.

1. _____

2. _____

3. _____

4. _____

5. _____

If you have more than five things you want from this book, go to the Note Pages at its back and write them there. Noting now what you want to get here sets your subconscious to be on the lookout for those points and zing you when it spots them. (Writing them also lets you check back after you finish the book to see if you got what you were looking for.)

If you don't, let me know! We'll include the additional info in the next book or our next blog article. If you want to know something that's not in here, it's for sure a lot of others are wanting the same thing; you can help them by letting us know what else is needed.

You may want to start a notebook for writing thoughts and feelings about topics we work on here. (I use inexpensive spiral bound notebooks to journal, on sale at Walmart and Target and KMart just before school starts . They're usually around twenty-five cents then. And you might want to get more than one of them.)

> **Psych Note:** Here's your payoff: This exercise jump-starts your subconscious mind to work for you. Getting clear about what you are looking for in advance primes your subconscious to be on the lookout and highlight them for you.

Whoops! It's Time to Eat a Frog!

A few years ago, John, one of my business mentors, taught me a new trick. Leaned toward me across the table, he said, "I've noticed that you have a problem with putting things off. Almost all of us have something every day a task on the to-do list that we don't want to do—that we hate even thinking about. And we all tend to put it off—as if putting it off will make it go away."

I had no trouble relating to what he was saying. Most of my to-do list consists of that kind of thing. I mean, if a task is easy or something I want to do, I don't need to put it on a list.

John, who makes no bones about anything, and is rarely concerned about whether his opinions might hurt your feelings, he speaks his truth—which is why I value him so much. Whimpering or sobbing with pleading eyes just rolls off him. (I've tried it.) So I just sat there that morning, waiting to see what he would say this time and wondering how awful it would be. And if I needed more coffee.

He began: "A speaker at a conference I recently went to gave some advice that has been one of the best pieces of business wisdom I've ever received. He said that you have to make a habit of selecting the most unpleasant task on your day's to-do list and do it first. ("Eeek!" I'm thinking. "He's going to ruin my life!") And he went on, paying no heed to my expression of displeasure.

"Getting that dreaded task done first," he said, "moves it out of the way—which means out of your mind. It's a heavy weight lifted and done with. Dealing with what you don't want to deal with ends up making you feel great. Now you don't have that heavy weight, and mental nagging that something awful is hanging over you and waiting for you.

"You think like a child when you put off ugly tasks. A part of you has a fantasy that the task will go away—or get less disgusting—if you put it off long enough."

Well, there I could see that he really was talking to me.

But some of those tasks do go away, I thought. Right—just after they shut off the electricity, or TV cable or . . . .

John was still going on. "This guy said, that he calls taking care of that kind of task 'eating a frog.' He said that most days you have tasks you enjoy, even look forward to, but also some you'd rather not do at all. However, if you are going to succeed at anything, you've gotta learn how to get those don't-want-to tasks done—like them or not.

"If not, they build a nest on your list and hatch out babies, he said, "byproducts of not taking care of the papa problem in time.

"In other words, tasks that you hate, if left undone, are guaranteed to create still more problems," he went on, "and you're going to hate them too. Probably worse."

"He said that most of us have to eat a frog every day. He also said that the reason he uses particular illustration is that if we eat a raw frog first thing, we can rest assured that nothing worse can possibly happen to us that day." We both laughed.

"Doing it first, you can relax and enjoy the rest of the day!"

And that brings us to you. Your frog for the day.

This frog is ugly, one you have imagined but couldn't bear to look at, one of the most unpleasant pieces of information I will give you in this book, so let's get it over with.

Chug it down. Hold still you slippery little pudgy devil!

And here's your awful news:

Once an over-drinker is past the earliest stages of an emerging drinking problem (which is long past if you're reading this book), his chances of turning it around are extremely slim.

Ah. There. Choke it down.

Yes, I know. Most of the hype you see on "cures" for alcoholism, alcohol abuse, problem drinking, or whatever the speaker calls it, give the idea that if you get the drinker into treatment, all will be well. But that just ain't so. Recovery has been made to sound like a reliable remedy. You can't help but pick up the idea that once you get him enrolled in treatment, all your trials are over. Voila! He'll come out a changed man. But that stereotype also isn't true.

The success of organizations such as Alcoholics Anonymous was so welcome after millennia of mankind's history fighting the drink that the world relaxed and rejoiced. Everyone got on the bandwagon for program-based treatment as a cure-all. Some of these cures seemed miraculous and much has been made of them—rightly so. But that caused people to see those cases as what usually happens. "Recovery" was received the way polio vaccine and antibiotics were, with gratitude and excitement. Expecting consistent high results.

We expected the alcohol problem fix to really fix them—so they stayed fixed—like a polio shot prevents ever getting polio, or an antibiotic cured pneumonia completely. Everyone was swept up in the hope that the relatively few lasting recoveries gave. They never told us that hundreds entered the "treatment" who never got it. What we have been shown are those who did.

Reality: Lasting recovery is the exception rather than the rule.

When you long for your man to change, you are longing for the wonderful guy you fell in love with. You may believe, from the hype, that this change will be complete, and there to stay. But it ain't so. My own research several years ago examining studies that used various methods of getting people sober, revealed that fewer than 10 percent of those trying to clean up will ever make it out and stay out. Perhaps more importantly for you is knowing this: Almost none will make the big effort to turn-around anytime soon.

This fact is extremely important for you because your fantasy is that he's going to have some kind of change, and soon—also that it will be complete and the man you fell in love with will return, never again to leave. And that fantasy must go.

Science and experience consistently show that once the downward cycle of over-drinking begins, changing the drinker's drinking will require a pile up of troubles and an incredible amount of pain to make that big first step of admitting—not only to you but to his innermost self—that he's in trouble and is now aware that he cannot stop and stay stopped.

All that required pain and trouble requires not only a very long time, but unacceptable pain and stress on everyone close to him. It won't happen quickly; it takes a long, long time, time filled with increasingly bad behavior, before he even wants to stop. And he must have help. He cannot do it on his own. Yes, you hear of such things happening, but after Early Stage, they include involvement in a church or some group that has the capacity to replace the drinking.

But that's not all: While it takes an over-drinker a very long time (years) to come to the point of admitting to himself that he's in big trouble, it will take even more time for him to admit to himself that he's going to need outside help to do it. (Over-drinkers are notoriously stubborn on this point, showing just how badly they are affected mentally. That's because it's not just the masculine tendency to want to be self-sufficient, it's his ego!) Only when he truly sees that others see, and that others know, will he begin to open up to his reality.

So after all those years of enduring him getting ever worse, the faint hope that "something" will happen is not nearly enough for a woman who is already hanging by a fragile thread, to hang her hopes on.

Even if you manage to get him to treatment, it's not likely to "take." (A couple of decades ago the word was in professional circles that an average of three passes through treatment were required for it to work. At how many thousands of dollars a pop? But we now know that for the majority, even that won't be enough.) Even if it "works," it is still precarious as to how long. Perhaps more importantly, the fact is that it's not likely to happen anytime soon.

You may be pushing yourself beyond human endurance (and to your own harm) in the belief you might soon get relief, that he might soon change. If only . . . . All the while, your body and mind continue to accumulate damage from stress inflicted on you as he runs his course to the bitter end. You're garnering more wounds. And aging. Prematurely, at that.

This isn't to say you need to separate. It is, however, saying that you can't keep surviving based on that hope. Bitter as is this truth, a drinker's woman must understand that the ability to make and continue with the gigantic changes required for an over-drinker to turn around bad drinking—and keep it that way—may already have been burned out of his brain.

Because of the damage to his brain's judgement center, it will take a long time for him to finally see that he has a problem. All the while, with every drink, he's getting worse, and your pressures continue to rise.

In the slim chance he gets to the point where he will go for help, and the even slimmer chance that the help he goes for actually helps, it will take still more time, usually years, for him to get close to being the man you dream of getting back.

Then, for that change to last more than a few days or weeks, he must spend the rest of his life working on rebuilding himself, work on getting new brain programming to replace what he's lost, work that cannot let up even for an hour. With all this and more required for him to have any hope of lasting success, understand that his change won't be something like waving a wand. I wish it would.

(The only research-proved successful treatment—which means the treatment that has the most lasting successes (still less than 10 percent) has been daily or almost daily gathering in groups of others like himself, groups such as in Alcoholics Anonymous where members teach each other, and strengthen each other. (All of this can sometimes be found in other groups with similar structure.) But to succeed, he must, absolutely must, work 24 hours a day, 365 days a year—with no let-up, guarding what he learns and gaining more ability, his own tricks, for strengthening the new things he must do to stay clean and sober.

Ugly fact: Even doing all that, only a small percentage of those who try will ever make it—and stay straight to the end of their lives.

If the drinker fails to do all these things—all these things—there is no chance that he can turn it around and keep it that way. If he lets up for even an hour, for all the rest of the years of his life, he will fall again. We see it continually, even after months and years of recovery.

If his chances of turning it around are so slim, if what seems like success still promise so little, then it makes no sense for you to tolerate the intolerable—in hope of turning him around. Disabusing you of this fantasy is my strongest reason for writing this book.

It's not so much staying with him that damages you, but staying with the fantasy that he'll change that will grind you down—and you are much too precious and rare a personality to allow that to happen. It is possible. however, for you to stay and, for some to create a satisfying life for themselves, but it will be separate from the life he will continue to drag down.

His slim chances of "recovery" don't mean you have to go; it only means you have to let go hanging on to the dream of him changing the way you want him to.

Now swallow it, this nasty frog. You must—in order to save yourself.

If you don't like it, it doesn't change a bit of what I've told you. It's truth, and only by understanding the truth can you save yourself. And have a miniscule chance of saving him.

Once you swallow this hideous froggy fact, you are going to start seeing everything differently. Your perspective changes, and not so much about him, but about yourself—your life, your future, how much more effort you are willing to put into trying to change him.

(Note: If lasting recovery were easy, your guy already would have made it. Most over-drinkers have actually tried

very hard, and many times (and they failed every time). So it's not for lack of trying—because he has. His problem is that he's like a golf wanna-be working to be a star, all the while insisting he doesn't need a golf club. His many attempts failed because he cannot do or think on his own what he must do and think in order to make it. He needs a "club.")

Good News: Already you better understand that his failure to beat the drinking isn't because he doesn't love you. It has nothing to do with how he does or doesn't you; he may try to make others believe it because that "gives him an excuse" for the way he drinks and treats you. He may still love you. But you must always remember that love just isn't enough! The behavior must change.

Behavior must reflect that love, must have a high priority on the welfare of his mate. (Then again, he may already have deteriorated far enough that he no longer is able to love—at least love anything more than he loves drinking.)

Over-drinkers often will say they love their woman; however, you must understand that love, the kind of love you long for, isn't just a feeling—it's a way of life. His ability to love is severely diminished by his inner changes, especially his brain changes. Love isn't just a feeling or words—love is the way you treat another person, day in and day out.

More Good News!

Cheer up, my beauties, I've found that rare is the swallowed frog that doesn't bring along some kind of blessing. The blessing attached to this particular frog is that once you take in the Bad News of your guy's reality, you gradually find yourself with a totally new understanding and outlook on what you're involved with. You have a new perspective—and it's going to make all the difference in your level of stability (and sanity).

Seeing things from a new perspective, all of a sudden, your hope of improving your own life can become reality.

You may occasionally think about what your life could be without all the discomfort, the dread, and stress, and emotional upset and pain. That daydream will become reality for you—whether he gets straightened out or not. I'm going to show you things that can make your life much easier—tricks to use, whether you decide to stay with him or separate.

The new tricks you'll be learning are going to give you much better control of how your days go. I've seen many women successfully remain in their homes and relationships by using these techniques. If you try staying but it doesn't work, you can always rethink the go-stay decision.

Face it: You have spent vast amounts of time and emotional energy obsessing on your problem—which is mostly him. You've tried to think up ways to get him to change—and sometimes he has. For the worse.

When the tactics you have used failed to accomplish needed changes, your reaction has been to try harder, spending hours of obsessing on coming up with a better plan. Most of you have repeated this cycle of try-something-fail-try-something over and over until it has become a way of life. Some of you can look at yourselves and realize you've become what you wouldn't have dreamed a few years ago. That's just no way to live.

It's time to decide, and you must decide soon so why not right now, that you are done with allowing his problem to dominate and damage your life, as it destroys his body and mind.

> **Psych Note:** An obsession is a thought or idea that returns despite your not wanting it to, or it interferes with your life. It's not an obsession if you enjoy thinking about it or if it doesn't interfere with your life. If you decide to stop, yet slip back to thinking the same thoughts, you've entered obsession. It can be overcome—and without medication in most cases. Some of the tricks—uh, techniques—that you'll soon be learning can also work well on dumping obsession.

* * *

Swallowing a Tadpole (In Comparison)

The next topic is a mere tadpole of ugly compared to the frog you just downed: Once he passes a specific point of brain cell death in his drinking—a point that can differs for different people (and which occurs much, much sooner than traditionally believed)—he will only get worse so long as he continues to drink any form of alcohol at all.

This makes sense: the alcohol starts damaging whatever was left from the last go-around that the body was unable to repair. His already damaged and unrepaired organs (especially his brain) now get the onslaught of a new dose of toxin. Thus, he continues to lose whatever brain power he had left.

At some point (again, much sooner than is currently accepted—in other words, we know it but "people" don't want to accept it) he no longer has the brain power to recover. It takes tremendous brain power to learn and do what is required.

Among other things, this means that it won't help for him to cut down, or to change from whisky to beer, or from beer to wine. It's the instantaneous action of alcohol on specific brain cells that turns off his ability to resist it.

The reason this awful truth is only a tadpole to deal with or swallow is its upside: Knowing in advance that his attempts to cut down (once he crosses his body's capacity to heal itself) won't work for long, you are set free. This ugly fact turns out to be slightly sweet. Here's why: Knowing it can relieve you of the tension, the stress of wondering if he'll come home drunk after promising to to be sober. You are already prepared for what is likely—he won't be alcohol-free. I can say this because my personal research into what few recovery rates are available indicate that fewer than 10 percent of those who attempt to quit can. And stay quit. That means 90 percent will drink and over-drink again. Thus, you are 90 percent sure he will eventually fall, so you are ready for it. No shattering surprise.

This means more than 90 per cent will eventually fail in these attempts. The relief here is in lifting the stress off you, the stress of watching, wondering, worrying if he'll have been drinking next time you see him. You can drop it now: You know there's practically no chance he will.

Let him try; give him your blessing; and quit stressing about him failing. You already know that it's almost certainly coming. And if it doesn't, if he is one of the 10 percent, that's wonderful! Only good can come from taking this mental position toward him.

In the meantime, don't let anything important hinge on his being sober at a specific time. Once you ease into the idea that he isn't likely to get better (and stay that way), you enter a new phase of existence. No longer spending mental energy worrying, or coming up with ways to get him to change. Picture what your life will be then. In fact, you'll actually have one!

You no longer need walk on eggshells. You no longer bother to sniff his breath. You no longer live in an unpredictable world, hinging on the slightest thing that might upset him. No more wondering if he's going to blow it; you already know he will.

This frees up all that time and energy to create for yourself a good life, with more fun in it—one with many more things to look forward to, many more things to do, and many more worthy accomplishments. Your new life will not focus on him but on fulfilling your personal goals and dreams and your children's. You can treat him kindly, and with respect—but you no longer obsess.

You can do all these things with or without him. Only you can decide which way is really best. If you get stuck, get some outside, uninvolved help to think it through; take your time. That is, only if he isn't violent. If he has ever been violent, jump to Chapter 9 right now. Then come back here.

Applying Your New Knowledge

Henceforth, you will not allow your plans or needs to depend upon his being sober or behaving appropriately. Since it's difficult for you to predict exactly when he will fall, the safest approach is to assume he may not be sober or behave well when you need him to.

That isn't disrespectful, it's reality—being quietly smart. All you need to do is create the habit of setting up a Plan B when his participation is part of any event.

Sound awful? Well, in fact, it makes things so much better that you'll soon be happy to take the few seconds to construct a Plan B where he's concerned. It's your road to freedom and peace of mind.

Always having a Plan B is one of the key tricks of living with an over-drinker. It may seem difficult at first, but so did your ABCs and learning to ride a bike. This new way of living comes fairly fast because most of the time it feels so much better.

In short time you hardly have to think about doing these new things—you just do them, When something feels good, it is rewarding. Your subconscious is a pig for "rewarding," and that sense of reward, allowing yourself to enjoy, even for a moment, accomplishing a new trick, is enough to do the job.

Your Good News is that your world doesn't have to fall apart if he does (fall apart).

Think about how you'd rather be: See yourself no longer anxious if he's late. (That's because you have a Plan B. Setting up an alternative method in case depending on him fails, taking care of yourself, getting into activities that are fun for you.)

Having Plan B means you'll rarely be thrown by some horrendous thing he does. You may even cease asking him to stop by to pick up Johnnie's birthday cake for the party—and if you must, you ask the bakery to phone you at a specific time if he hasn't shown up, a time that will allow you to send someone else.

This trick teaches you not to don't count on his being sober for an event. You, unruffled, will put your Plan B into operation, get dressed and go out to a fine gathering yourself. Simply explain to others that he's not well, then go on and have a great time. (Most others already know—long before you think they do—that he's got a problem with drinking.)

On those occasions, he probably won't be a problem by the time you get back. He will be totally drunk and passed out—which you also now begin to see as another plus, another new perspective. And he enjoys because he can switch from feeling guilty and humble to being enraged and haughty because you went without him.

A warning: Many women have made the mistake of believing that a falling-down drunk couldn't hurt them—or that if he passed out that they would be safe for a time. Both of those ideas are dead wrong. A falling down drunk can still kill without and never remember any of it.

Some women, believing that they were safe after their man passed out, were killed when he suddenly rose and caught them trying to leave.

An over-drinker who has passed out can suddenly become alert, instantly enraged, and leap up to kill. This is one of the oddities of alcohol's affect on the disintegrating brain.

To get started reducing your stress, keep always in mind the following two tidbits:

1. There is *no* way to please a person who can't be pleased. Bearing in mind that he will rarely be satisfied with anything—his feel-good comes to work only when he's drinking. Expect him to be dissatisfied and complain and criticize; don't hang onto the hope that this time will be different from all the other times. Believing that he will be satisfied if only you get it right this time sets you up for a big let-down. It's okay to drop the wearying stress of trying to do things "right" (which means "his way"). Besides, you already know "his way" is subject to rapid change—without notice.

Solution: You cease doing anything in the hope he'll be satisfied if you just get it "right." Especially if you're never quite sure what "right" is going to be at any given time.

2. He is wholly invested, totally determined to come out on top, and at almost any cost.

He has more than a tinge of nutsy in this area. However, knowing this, you won't invest much in a discussion or endeavor involving him. Your life will get sweeter if you will let him come out on top—in his own mind at least—whenever possible. (Keep in mind that he loves to make you look stupid so he can dismiss what you think, specially about his drinking!) Just resign from arguing anything with him. That doesn't mean give up, because on most points you can do as you please anyway. For the rest, keep in mind the mental and emotional price of arguing with him.

* * *

Diane Talks With Us
(Note: Diane is a made-up name, as are all others used in this book, accompanied by a skewed description. That way these wonderful women stay anonymous.)

I meet Diane in the front room of my office and she comes with me into the counseling room. Ripples of sun flow through the thin curtains, bringing a pleasant light in here. I love this room. Thirty-ish, attractive, Diane is as tense as most people are on their first visit here. She accepted the coffee I offered and was already enjoying, and we settled in. I began getting basic information from her that we need to get a better understanding of how some problems may have formed. Just knowing that doesn't cure the problem, but usually, knowing how a problem formed holds keys to remedies.

I pulled out my intake forms, and she answered the basic questions easily. I could see her begin to relax through the process; indeed, we were getting to know each other in the easy talk—the basics. But she lost her comfort when I reached the part asking about her reasons for wanting to come see me.

Her posture and facial expression tensed, she stiffened slightly in the chair as she fidgeted in the chair, her eyes shifting from me to the windows and various corners of the room. Her tension and discomfort signaled that along with whatever else she brought in, it was wrapped in a strong dose of anxiety. She was signaling that she was afraid of the topic she wanted to address. My job was to help her feel safer.

A moment passes. She takes a deep breath and begins, her voice strengthening as she begins to speak, her body relaxing.

"To tell you the truth, I really came to see you because I think I'm going crazy."

"Well, let's see if that's true," I say. "That's pretty easy to determine! It's not a dark secret to tell whether someone's really crazy," I say with a grin. It works, Diane shakes her shoulders and relaxes slightly. "So talk to me about you, about things you've noticed that have caused you to worry about going crazy."

"Well, I'll tell you about me in general first. I'm married, have two children, Melissa is 12 and Tony is 10. I'm an assistant to the Vice President of XX bank, not a secretary so much as a general assistant in all areas. I believe I'm very good at what I do," she says. Part of why I'm here has to do with my children." She stops, appears distracted, distraught.

"Both of them have changed, and neither one in a good way. I'm really worried about what to do, but nothing I've tried so far is helping much. Maybe the real thing I'm coping with is feeling helpless, and stressed too, like I'm going to explode sometimes, but that has mostly to do with my husband Bob." She stops, looks directly at me and adds, "I haven't been copying well with his attitude and actions lately."

"How about you give me an example of some of the things you mean, the kind of things you don't think you are reacting well to," I say.

"He used to be fun, cuddly—and now it's all I can do to get him to stay home—or even speak to me in a respectful way."

She stops, leans back, pauses, looks away. "He's become so ugly, saying the meanest things—to me, especially, but also to the kids." She pauses. Several seconds pass.

"He's hardly ever home any more. He says he's working, but I know that a lot of what he calls 'work' goes on in the bar after hours. He's drinking a lot more at home too." She sighed. "I don't know if he's having an affair, and I'm coming to thinking that would be great—just to keep him out of the house even more.

"Another thing worrying me is that I'm forgetting things—things I need to remember, like what my boss asks me to take care of, things I need to do for the kids, doctor appointments. I don't know if the stress at home is getting to me, or if I'm losing my mind." She suddenly leans back into the chair as if all the air has gone out of her with her words.

Now we began to explore specifics, such as what type of things she was forgetting, and when she did it most—and the best she could remember of what else was going on at the same time. As we dug into this area, she straightened up and said, "You know, it happens a lot right after an argument! And the next day or so too," she added thoughtfully. The energy, the joy that insight brings accompanies even bad discoveries in therapy; I saw the signs now.

(This happens because correctly identifying the "bad" things, the problems, is key to fixing them. That's why therapists dig into your past and current life—most "bad" things you encounter in the present have grown from seedlings planted long ago, usually when you were very young.

"Tell me a bit more about those arguments, and also some more details about his drinking," I say. She ran down a list of events that clearly showed he was drinking too much (pretty much the same list hundreds of women have brought to me before Diane.)

I probed a few of the things she told me, and smiled: "I think we have something that just might help you," I said, pulling out a copy of the questionnaire you'll be getting in Chapter 5. It's a guide to examining a drinking problem. I asked her to wait to work on it until she could get an hour or so of alone time— "which, it sounds like, you are having more of lately, so let's use it positively—for your benefit!" I added.

After getting more details from her, I told her about some of the positive personality qualities I had already seen in her—her courage, her intelligence, her concern for others, her willingness to work hard for goals, her capacity to forgive or lay aside some pretty upsetting behavior for a greater good. And more. All these are qualities I can almost guarantee that you too possess.

Diane was intrigued when I told her that the personality traits I was ticking turn out to be common to all the women who have ever come to me for help and who had men who drank too much.

"But there's something wrong with me," she said. I need to know what you see is wrong. My friends tell me that I'm just too good. Too giving, too forgiving—too nice! It's confusing to think those are good things about me.

(Note: All drinkers's women are in need of knowing who they really are. Not being aware of their true beauty, and being continually criticized will cause anyone to begin to doubt and mistrust themselves.)

"I don't much like myself at all," Diane adds. "I can see that I really am a big part of the problem. He says that often enough..

"I've become a nervous wreck trying to do everything right so he won't get upset, go on a rampage. I know the things he hates, but I manage to do them anyway—like he says, it's like I'm asking for it, for him to blow up at me," slumping, pausing. "I've about given up on myself; I'm all out of things to try to fix me, and to get him to do what he should, to just be more of a husband and dad.

"He says our problems are because of the way I do things, but no matter how hard I work to get things the way he wants, there's always something."

She pauses, looks out the window, she seems to relax after just shedding what must have been a tremendous weight.

Me: "I'm so glad that you've come to me, Diane. I believe you may have a problem that happens to be one of my areas of expertise! I've had many, many years of experience in working with this problem.

"Some of what you say is beginning to sound familiar. Let me ask you a couple of questions to get a better understanding, okay?"

"Sure," she said.

I proceeded to ask the same questions I ask every women who brings in a problem similar to Diane's, and she began giving me the same answers so many others have brought in.

I told her about a trait that most drinkers's women have and that she had in a mega-dose—her willingness to accept responsibility for her errors, and do whatever she knew to fix them. That's a beautiful quality, unless (like most other things in life) it's overdone. Another trait I pointed out to her was her determination to take care of her family's problems—all alone if necessary, with no partner as was meant to be for raising a family. And she had been doing all that while carrying on all her other task and working a full-time jobs. These observations point out her true strength, not the fact that she—like an elephant of camel—will break down when the load is too great. A partner who is steadily criticizing, beating her down, intentionally or not.

"It's the behavior he chooses now, how he behaves, that is doing the damage," I tell her, "and the behavior currently stressing you is what you focus on instead of the man, the man you once knew.

"You definitely are suffering the effects of stress, Diane, and it's reaching a worrisome level. If what I think is going on really *is* going on, you're going to be amazed at how simple, even easy, your next steps are going to be. Take this booklet and try to scan through it; and," as I pulled out more papers from a file, "I'd like for you to work on these this week so we have a lot more to go on from here. If anything here puzzles you or gives you trouble, call the office and I'll get back to you as soon as possible. You shouldn't have a problem, but if you do, I'm here.

"We're almost out of time, so I would like to know what your questions are right now, that you'd like answered before we set up another appointment. What else you need to know to move forward? To feel more comfortable over the next week as you keep thinking about what we're talking about now. I want you to pay as much attention to what you have said as you pay to what I have said. Sound okay for you?"

"Gosh," she said, looking at the papers, "I'm so full of new information now, I can't think of anything else I need."

"That's good," I said. "If burning questions arise, just give me a call and we'll talk again before next week. Okay?"

"Yes, that's great. I think I'm going to get a lot more from working on these papers you've given me. Thank you so much; I know it's not all well, but I really feel so much better—just talking to someone who really understands all this," she said .

"Diane," I said, "it is my joy to work with such an intelligent and lovely woman."

"Thank you," she said, "can I see you next week at this same time?" she asked.

"Let me look at the appointment book," I said, going into the reception area and opening the book. "Yep, looks like next week is open at this time too. Looks like we're off to a good start."

* * *

So—here we are: Chapter One is coming to an end. You've taken in a lot of information. Four important ideas from this chapter I'd like for you take away are these:

1. The over-drinker has only the slimmest chance of ever turning around his drinking problem—and keeping it that way.
2. If he drinks any alcohol at all, he'll keep getting worse.
3. If he tries to quit, he will almost certainly fail. (Knowing that helps you stabilize your own life despite what he does—as best you can at any given moment.)
4. His bad behavior has created multiple, serious stressors for you—and it has broken your heart. This means you've picked up a load of emotional and mental harm. Fortunately, with the right approach, it's quite fixable! I've worked with hundreds of women who all eventually grasp enough of these ideas to begin living an interesting, rewarding life.

Okay, my lovelies, we end our first session.
So far, you're doing great!
Now—Down the hatch with all these slippery little suckers, frogs, tadpoles, and all!
Ahhh . . . So long, Froggy.
So long, Tadpoles.
Hello, Silver Lining!

Oh, one more thing:
Take my word for this, babe: It ain't you that's the problem!

Got Coffee? Tea?

I'm writing to you as if we're talking face to face—in my office, in a lovely park, or sitting under a large umbrella on the beach. (We make therapy as much fun as we can!)

Why don't you go fetch yourself something nice to sip—coffee or cola, herbal tea or fruit juice—whatever enhances your relaxed reading—and settle down here with me for a while longer.

* * *

Chapter 2

Where you
 Find out whether it's just you!
 Learn tricks for side-stepping ugly moments
 Find out when you definitely must lie!

Bad Behavior? Let Us Count the Ways!

Who's the Real Victim of a Drinking Problem?

Our society calls the drinker "the victim" of the alcohol disorder. Indeed, he is a victim; his genetics, something he can do nothing about, are what likely set him up to enter a very real hell once he began over-drinking. But the disorder injures others as badly as he is injured, often worse emotionally, and they would be the people who live with him. When drinking goes bad, it becomes the only disorder where the afflicted person has fun (he thinks) while the people around him suffer, get sick, and are emotionally wounded, frequently scarred for life.

Overwhelming stressors confront those close to an over-drinker, but the bulk of the stress the drinker generates falls on his woman. After all, who is closest to the action?

Who has to take up the slack when he's unwilling or unable? Who gradually comes to have to do the job of two for the family? Who must try to pay bills, run a household, parent children—on diminished funds and with precious little help? Who is humiliated when the drinker is publicly inappropriate? And when he doesn't remember what he did, whom does he accuse of lying when she tries to tell him about it? Who struggles to explain the unexplainable to children, parents, friends? Many of whom will disagree and say something like, "He's not that bad!"

And who has to cover for him—even taking the blame for things herself to keep the bad actor in the clear?

Whose home life, social life, family life, personal life, mental and emotional wellbeing are severely affected by the over-drinker's unpredictable emotional storms and behavior?

Some will even blame her for his drinking! ("Can't blame him, she's such a nag.")

So who? Right, it's his woman. You.

Well, hold on, girl. You can change much of the outfall from his drinking once you understand what's happening to him, and get some guidance on how to more successfully make changes.

After the Early Stage, an over-drinker's drinking and the behavior it begins to produce start affecting his life in many areas. How many areas affected is a good measure of how far the disorder has progressed. To get a basic idea of your guy's situation, check any areas affected in your man's life by his drinking (which includes anything associated with his drinking).

___ Home life ___ Family relationships
___ Social life ___ Financial standing
___ Family life ___ Sex Life
___ Mental and emotional wellbeing

If someone's drinking negatively affects any—any—of their life areas, and the drinker doesn't stop drinking, it is sufficient evidence to diagnose a drinking disorder.

In Chapter 5, you'll find a detailed list of the numerous signs of a drinking disorder, a list that I've created to demonstrate that there are masses of signs that someone is in trouble with his drinking long before he is currently diagnosed (and treated).. With this expanded list of signs of problem drinking, countless lives will be saved, the lives of both drinkers and their women.

Yet, even with all those signs in Chapter 5, there is a single sign that is never wrong. This sign of serious trouble is when his drinking starts interfering with his life and he doesn't stop.

Let's look at some of the ways your guy's drinking has affected your life. Go down the same list of life areas that his drinking has affected—and check any of them in your life that his drinking has affected.

___ Home life ___ Financial Standing
___ Social life ___ Sex life
___ Family Life ___ Mental and Emotional
___ Family relationships   wellbeing

How many of his life areas did you check? _____ (of 7)
How many of your life areas? _____ (or 7)

You are aware that his behavior has affected you, but are you aware of how seriously they have affected you. In fact, many of the effects on you of stress caused by *his* drinking, you have blamed yourself for. Cracking is the result of an outside force hammering in; the cracked egg isn't weaker than other eggs.

(Note: You likely demand of yourself to tolerate the intolerable. I have never met a woman who was not severely affected by her partner's over-drinking after not very long. The over-drinker's behavior gradually impacts his woman. Because "cracking" occurs with all over-drinkers's women, it's time to dump your tendency to down yourself for it. You believe downing yourself will make you do better, but it doesn't; it makes you do worse. Practices that you have believed are good for you—fussing at yourself, looking for a weakness in yourself when things go wrong—is good only in small doses for people in normal situations. But when you live with an over-drinker, it's a boon—to him. The drinker will go to almost any lengths to make himself look good, not being the bad guy or having a problem. Thus he protects his ability to drink. He is skilled in "suggesting" that others are to blame. He blames the city his bad mood for having to stop at red lights to justify his rage and ranting.)

You do not deserve the discomfort and emotional pain of being blamed or blaming yourself. Still, the only part of that you can control is what you do to yourself—usually at his suggestion that the fault is yours. The habit of looking for your flaws, as well as the habit of taking what he says about you as truth, began long ago and likely far away from him. It just happens to be your willingness to look at your own mistakes to correct them, that originally set you up to become a drinker's woman.

You can't sweep away that habit; you *can* replace it. When you catch yourself fussing at yourself (cussing yourself?), immediately remind your inner critic of at least one of your truly good traits or skills.

Most people in therapy find that the voice of what they thought was their inner critic is actually the voice of a parent. Work on this with friends—perhaps form a group dedicated to helping each other dump their harsh criticism of themselves. Losing it for good begins with understanding where you learned to think that way, and why you took it up as a habit.

For starters, list on the next page some of the ways that you might have learned this habit?

What was it that made you begin doing it so often that it became a habit? The true cause is going to be something good about you.

So how and why would you say you learned to demand the impossible from yourself?

It's easiest said in this form: I learned to fuss at myself by taking in what significant others said about me; I learned to fuss at myself because I wanted to please those significant others; I wanted approval; I wanted to avoid disapproval. All of the above.

_____

_____

For many of you, it also was to avoid punishment. "Punishment" includes seeing (or believing) that the other person rejects the total you because of a misdeed.

Hating rejection is wired in to the human brain. It's a survival mechanism, not a flaw. It's in us to guard our position in the group and that's because we survive best in groups.

To feel rejected when parents find something in you to protest is not so harmful as when parents were sure to let you know that you were on the black list. I have found that most drinkers's women were treated as if they were unloved when they erred. The child's sense of losing love because of making a mistake makes a great impression. The withdrawal of love, dependent on one's behavior, creates a kink in the personality. That individual will either go to any lengths to gain approval, or will throw off all restraints and lose respect for the punishers.

If the rejection, especially the withdrawal of love, is repeated, it creates a deeper drive to please. In many, it leads to rejecting the reject-ers. For some of them it goes into full rebellion. If any of this applies to you, and it will to most, you must go outside yourself for healing. Good friends who are savvy to these ideas, or a group, or a counselor are your most effective healers.

Knowing that his drinking and the behavior it causes have damaged your relationship, you also know that you've been frustrated and hurt by the things he does and says—his behavior. But you may not have been aware until now of how powerfully those effects have begun to change you, and not for the better. One harmful force is the deterioration of your relationship. The following list contains some of the effects other drinkers's women have reported. Few of you will have experienced them all, but all drinkers's women have experienced most.

Commonly Reported Effects of Women Once Their Mate Begins Over-Drinking
(Check any of these you've already experienced.)

1. ____ Losing time with your partner that you used to enjoy.
2. ____ Losing the sense you are his most important interest.
3. ____ Losing the feeling of being a big part of his life.
4. ____ Feeling left out.
5. ____ Feeling inadequate as a partner.
6. ____ Feeling you're not attractive enough.
7. ____ Worrying about your partner's waning interest.
8. ____ Losing trust in your partner.
9. ____ Not feeling the sweet bond you used to feel.
10. ____ Feeling he doesn't care about your needs.
11. ____ Worrying about what's happening to your dreams or plans.
12. ____ Worrying about why you don't do things together anymore.
13. ____ Spending time and energy trying to change things.
14. ____ Feeling hurt or frustrated when things you try change don't.
15. ____ Losing the strength and confidence in life that your relationship once gave you.
16. ____ Feeling alarmed as you see him lose good parts of his personality, such as his intelligence, his integrity, even his sense of humor.
17. ____ Losing the fun in your relationship.
18. ____ Losing fun and romance in your sex life.
19. ____ Losing joy in things that you used to enjoy.
20. ____ Worrying about your partner's safety.
21. ____ Worrying about your future, your stability.
22. ____ Your frustration and dwindling trust often block closeness.
23. ____ Being embarrassed by his behavior.
24. ____ Putting your dreams and goals on hold while you wait for "things" (him) to stabilize.
25. ____ Your natural needs are not being adequately filled.

Let's stop here and examine human needs. Many of you have picked up the idea that having needs is a sign of being weak or mentally unstable, yet all of your true needs were wired in by an all-knowing Manufacturer. You are not flawed if you have needs; you are perfect! You have needs, again, to insure your survival.

When your needs go unfulfilled, it weakens you, you feel confused, anxious, depressed. Unmet needs create mental tension, and the stress that unmet needs produce can worsen an existing illness or create one.

On the next list, I want you to check any of your (completely normal) emotional needs not being *adequately* filled at this time.
(Note: "Adequately filled" means that you feel good, secure comfortable and fulfilled in that area of yourself. Just getting a little bit of fulfillment is NOT "adequately filled.")

1. Yes or No   Is your need for affection being filled?
2. Yes or No   Is your need for companionship being filled?
3. Yes or No   Is your need for respect being filled?
4. Yes or No   Is your need for a sense of belonging being filled;
5. Yes or No   Is your need to feel competent being filled?
6. Yes or No   Is your need to feel of worth, of value, being filled?
7. Yes or No   Is your need to be appreciated being filled?
8. Yes or No   Is your need to give love, and to be loved, to feel loved, being filled?

How many of these eight items got a "No" answer? _____

Now consider: Do the results of this inventory add to your understanding of what's been going on with you?   Yes or No

> **Psych Note:** All healthy people have all these listed needs. Their purpose is to keep you alive and well, physically, mentally, emotionally, and spiritually.

When under stress, you need more fulfillment in these areas in order to restore balance; if these needs continue to be unmet they create ever increasing stress. Your body and mind know that the whole of you is in danger and they are reacting be prodding you, which you feel as stress. Unfulfilled needs are why you get cranky or blue—far more often than your hormones cause distress. Having unmet needs is like driving a car without filling its needs! It struggles on gamely for a while, but then it dies.

You wouldn't expect a machine to do without what it needs to function. And when a machine stops running well, then just stops running, do you think it is a weakness in the machine itself, or do you think that something it needs to run right is missing? The problem is that your specific machine likely is not having its specific needs met. Yet most of you are embarrassed, ashamed, to have or show these needs. What's wrong with that picture?

Well, of course! If you think that having needs is due to inadequacy, or being flawed, something's drastically wrong with your use of the wiring necessary for survival.

Has anyone tried to make you feel ashamed because you have these needs? Called you needy—or worse? Yet all healthy people have these needs. Even animals have them.

After learning this about your personal needs, you will no more allow anyone to say (or imply with a look) that you are abnormal or inferior because you have them. It's not having them that's abnormal.

The normal response to unfulfilled emotional needs is that they begin to scream louder and louder to be filled—just as your physical needs do when you are hungry or thirsty or need to go to the bathroom. The longer those needs are unfulfilled, the more demanding they become. They don't let up if you try to ignore them, and they certainly don't go away if they aren't filled.

Don't think that because some few persons have lived under such harsh conditions that all of their needs became petrified, that is in any way the norm. We were created to love, and to be loved, to care about others and their welfare, and we are also wired to care for ourselves. You possess all these qualities—some of the most important to mankind's survival. Without these wired-in functions, humans become destructive and greedily violent.

Do you still think you should close down those emotional needs in yourself? To close them down is to turn yourself into a zombie, the walking dead. The life is all gone out of you.

Having unmet emotional needs causes you to lose your joy in life, to lose physical and mental energy, to become listless, distracted, unfocused, forgetful, irritable—especially toward yourself.

Whew! No wonder you've been out of sorts lately!

Living creatures—puppies, ponies, pollywogs, and people—whose basic emotional needs are not met, all end up either trying to numb or shut down those needs (as they scream ever louder), or seeking substitutes to fill their spaces. (Substitutes can be over-drink yourself, or over-medicating the inescapable anxiety or depression, over-eating, excitement-seeking, such as gambling and sexual adventures, or its opposite—over-sleeping and killing your desire for sex.

Unmet emotional needs cause one to gradually become a zombie; it's when a woman tries to heal her pain by turning off, denying her personal needs. Or she becomes needy and clingy. And always—she is angry.

Is there any Good News here? Yes, ma'am: At least you now understand much of what's been happening to you.

Let's See What Your Checklist Answers Suggest

Now go back to the checklist on changes in your relationship that you worked on earlier. How many checkmarks did you make on it? _____

Here's a "rough" assessment of what your numbers suggest about how his drinking and associated behaviors are affecting you.

One or Two Checkmarks

A score of one or two indicates that either the drinker doesn't yet have a real drinking problem—or he's just getting started. (If he does have a problem, your number of checkmarks will soon increase.)

> **Psych Note:** Here's Good News! Especially for those of you whose men are just beginning to ramp up their drinking. In the Early-Early Stage you can still talk to him, point out specifics of the problems coming from the drinking (but keep it to one, maybe two at a time or he'll shut out what you say). Tell him fully their negative effect on you.
>
> For a few drinkers, in the earlier Early Stages, creating awareness of how he affects you (and use words like "hurt," "afraid," "unhappy," "miserable." Use emotional words to describe what his drinking is doing to you.
>
> For a few Early Stagers, it can work. While that is quite rare,

> nevertheless, it can, and that makes it worth trying, a few times.) Changing his awareness of the consequences of his drinking (you can include any bad effects it's already having on other areas of his life here for greater impact, but keep that to only one or two also.)

The drinker is unlikely to accept that he may already be in trouble. If things aren't too bad, he has little motivation strong enough to stop. He doesn't see that he is racing into a physical condition so severe it will first rob, then destroy him and those around him. Always, always keep in your mind that, while he may have had a spot of trouble, the feeling he gets when he drinks is so wonderful that it outweighs the discomfort he has suffered so far—and the very vague threat (in his mind) it will get worse.

So long as he drinks anything at all, this will always be the way he thinks. The here-and-now reward of a drink is more powerful, carries more weight, than thoughts of what he considers "maybe" harm. Early Stage, when he has his best chance of fixing it, gradually slipping or exploding into Middle Stage.

Those drinkers whom alcohol makes especially good (mostly due to their inherited body makeup—especially brain, liver, kidney, pancreas and chemistry) are not as likely to respond even in the earliest phases. The feeling they get is so powerfully wonderful to them that they are practically hooked from their earliest experiences—even if they turn out to get them in trouble. The one thing that current treatment does not address is a separation of these varied body types—the importance is prime. That's because the effective cure will be different for each of the types. And stages.

Once treatment implements these protocols, success rates will rise.

I have come to have little or no confidence in the big money that creates and runs formal treatment. It's going to take large numbers of well educated counselors and therapists, with many more of them having experienced and lived recovery (and the hell that preceded it). These therapists should have at least a master's degree in either addictions or psychology, and several licensed psychotherapists on staff for difficult case handling and training of counselors-therapists, and for doing actual therapy. All of that takes money—and for the money currently being paid for treatment, it can be done.

My experience has been that directors of these programs pull down huge salaries, while the people on the front lines are paid barely above minimum wage. That's just one point where better use of available funding could begin

The sad part I've seen in most treatment over at least the last 40-plus years (and I have worked in almost every form of it) is that "counselors" may have no formal education at all. Too many of those who do have a degree have it in a field unassociated with psychology or counseling. A bachelor's degree in math or business is useless for dealing with a broken soul filled with self-hatred and rage, and screaming inside for the only thing that has ever brought him relief. Therapists prepared with those educations throw up their hands and tell the family the drinker "just isn't ready yet" when he returns to drinking after treatment. We have some terribly messed-up minds here, and the closer you look at what is called "treatment," the clearer you see why it hasn't been working so well.

Other research (reported by Harvard Medical School) found that those receiving treatment and then staying sober, almost to a man, immediately pick up going to AA meetings as soon as they leave treatment—and stay with it for the rest of their lives.

Likewise, the same study found that those who do not make it, almost to a man, did not take hold of the only thing we have to date that works at all—which has been Alcoholics Anonymous, and its record isn't very good if you want somebody to get sober and stay sober.

None of what I'm writing disparages those counselors who have poured their very lives into the work of helping alcoholics find and maintain sobriety. They are like you in being of the very best of God's creatures; they live to give to others. What I disparage is the corporations behind modern "treatment," and their structure and goals of these businesses, businesses whose primary aim is to make money. And they do.

Five to twenty years of over-drinking and deranged behavior can lie between this Early Stage opportunity for change and the next, the End Stage—when the next-best door of escape appears. That's when he will cry for help, and when others will finally force him to get it. Sadly, even then, only a handful will make it out—and stay out (due mostly to the loss of brain power caused by the corrosive effects of alcohol).

Here's the worst part: By the time he can get (and agrees to)

treatment, you will be five to twenty years older.

You may no longer have the strength to pull out either.

Three to seven checkmarks

signify that his drinking has been blasting holes in your relationship—and your life. By this point, the over-drinker will have begun occasionally trying to cut down. Or stop. But he always slips back. (Let me warn you too: Frequently, after an attempt to stop, a drinker will start up again and his drinking will now reach a more destructive level than when he stopped.

(Note: Contrary to common thought, until End Stage, over-drinkers are quite good at stopping. Stopping is not their problem! They do it frequently. "Quitting is easy," recovering drinkers will say, "I've done it a hundred times.")

No, his problem, the thing he cannot do, is *stay* stopped.

In the Early Stage of developing a problem, the over-drinker can't accept that anything that feels so good is hurting him. From the start all the way to End Stage, he's mostly having what he calls fun. As he's becoming addicted, he sees no reason to stop.

He can't see how bad it's getting, and he ignores any glimpses because he wants (very soon begins to need) the feelings alcohol brings him. Understanding this, you may understand (not approve of) why he gets hostile if you suggest he should quit.

He begins to see anyone trying to stop him from "having fun" as the enemy. He thinks, "They don't want me to have any fun!"

The man developing a drinking problem will try innumerable times to cut down or quit, and the most of these attempts he will keep to himself. In Middle Stage, likely most every morning he will vow to himself to stop—and be unable to stop from getting that early beer, or lunch cocktail, and not understand or believe that shoots him out of the cannon again. He feels so horribly miserable, physically and mentally, and he only knows one thing that can ease it. Guess what that is.

He stops telling others about his vows because he has failed so many times in past attempts that he has no confidence that he can make it this time either and doesn't want to be embarrassed again.

All of this explains how you may notice he's not drinking, or drinking less—for a time (usually quite short a time). You can take that behavior as confirmation that he has already tried many times, and failed. Now he doesn't want to spotlight his weakness by having (or the threat of having) others see another failure.

It also means he expects to fail. While means he's in Middle or Late Middle Stage of deterioration.

When a drinker who has begun drinking too much (over-drinking) occasionally succeeds at cutting down or stopping for any period of time—even three days—a weird twist of his mind leads him to believe that just because he could quit at all, he can't possibly have a drinking problem!

That's the height of "magic" thinking. It's a form of denial.

Worse, much of the rest of the world believes it too.

In this, he thinks he is reclaiming his manhood. We know he saw his drinking becoming a problem; that's what made him want to cut down or quit in the first place. So he knows. At least a part of him knows.

But he thinks being able to quit means he's okay, still manly—that doesn't have a problem! (Serial murderers can quit for a while too, for Pete's sake.) Nail-biters can quit for a while, shop-a-holics, dieters. All these things have much in common. Just as many women (me included) develop around menopause vast cravings for chocolate and other sweets, and we struggle with vowing to change—and failing, so he battles, with only one difference: What he craves is busily eating away his brain, like termites in sweet lumber—that brain which is his only hope of finding a way to quit. And stay quit.

You know that just stopping anything for a while doesn't mean the problem has gone away. Or never existed, as many over-drinkers will claim. They will say their ability to stop for a week, a month, even a year, is proof they really don't have a problem. But that's not true.

Alcoholics Anonymous offers the test that never fails. Get an over-drinker to drink one—only one—drink every day for 30-60 days without missing a day, or ever drinking more than one drink.

A problem drinker cannot do this. Many will say, "Well, I'll just quit," but that doesn't prove that their brain is affected by the elixir. Proof is being able to drink just one small drink, one small beer, one five-ounce glass of wine every day for at least 30 days and not do a drop more. Or less.

Most opt to quit because there's nothing quite as horrible as taking one drink and having that buzzing bee turn on, because it is only minutes before he calls in the whole hive. It is a living hell because of what happens in a damaged brain when new alcohol flips its switch. It is hell because it is all-consuming and you cannot escape it. You cannot even think of what to do instead.

But a problem drinker (99 percent of them) believes that stopping for days or even weeks means the problem is "all gone." Worse, they even believe it means they never had a problem in the first place. But don't let them fool you ever again with this weird thinking. It isn't true: In fact, stopping his drinking is a proof that it is a problem, or he would have no reason to stop it.

Don't be shy about sharing this with others! The point: Over-drinkers can quit. They just can't stay quit.

Believing his own erroneous conclusion, he crows about his two days, two weeks, or two months that he quit or cut down (to convince anyone within earshot that he doesn't have a problem). Of course, you might ask yourself "What normal drinker would do that?") Those announcements are a dead give-away that you're dealing with a man who is already caught in the alcohol trap.

The up-side to his failure at cutting down or quitting is that it proves some important points for you: It proves 1) that at some level he is aware of what's wrong. You know that because he decides he needs to quit drinking. This wouldn't occur to a normal drinker.

More Good News: His crowing behavior also shows that a part of him is fully aware of both the problem—and its cure. His subconscious knows in living color that what's causing his problems.

It's the drinking. **And his subconscious also knows the cure: The proof is that he decides to stop the drinking!**

But knowing isn't doing. His mistake (and that of most people) is believing that a drinking problem is like a cold—after it gets better, you're all well. Wrong! The failure of maintaining the cut-down drinking, or stay stopped is proof that he has already lost control of his drinking.

He couldn't stay away from it. He went back. He couldn't stop (and stay stopped) when he wanted to. This is what is meant when you say he has lost control: He can no longer do what he wants to do; the drinking calls, then controls him.

When he starts up again after cutting down, he will likely try to hide it from you. At first. Expect that he will try to get you to agree that it's okay. "I've done good, Baby, so just one won't hurt, will it?" You: "I guess not. But only one, you hear!"

And Blam! We're on the slippery slide again.

Here's Good News: Even when he tries to hide his failure to stay stopped, if he sneaks drinks and you miss it—no sweat! If he gets by with it once, there is no force on earth that will keep him from taking the next drink. It may be now, tomorrow, next week, or two weeks from now. But it's coming. Just sit back and relax; let go of the worry. We already know he's going to fail. And then, the next day, the next week, remember that he is saying to himself: "Gee, I didn't have any trouble when I drank a beer last week. I'm well."

Then, after he gets away with one drink a time or two, you must understand that nothing—not prison, not being tied down in a sanitarium, not your threats to leave him—nothing—will prevent his taking another drink at some point in the near future.

That's because he, and you, believe the problem is in how much he drinks, the amount he drinks. Once you understand that the slightest bit of alcohol fires up brain connections and his desire for more, you realize that he will start up again.

He can put it off (in the Early Stages), but it's just a matter of time until he breaks, follows his urge, his desire, his craving. Nevertheless, you now no longer sweat whether he's sneaking, nipping. You've stopped worrying, stopped sniffing his breath. stopped seeking out his hiding places, calling or driving to check up on where he really is. You now relax because know in advance that once he takes that first drink, he'll shortly be getting more.

And once drinking begins causing problems, it will always cause problems. Once it breaks through the brain's defenses, they are forever broken. They . . . do . . . not . . . grow . . . back!

In appropriate treatment, he will learn new tricks, come to understand he can't rely on tricks that have let him down 100 times. But he's not there now. He still believes he has the power to straighten up. But he doesn't.

(As to "the first drink," successful people in recovery are taught and listen to the truth: It's the first drink that gets them drunk! The rest of the world raises their eyebrows at this because the rest of the world still wrongly judges drinking problems by how much one drinks. It's hard to change that thinking, but you must. As you have just been reading, the reality of addiction, of craving, is that once he breaks and takes even a single drink, it swipes out every bit of "will power" or whatever it is that he was building. Once that's done, he's left weaker, and his inner drives are all focused solely on getting more. And that occurs quite early on in the development of a drinking problem—not in the last stages as most of the world believes.)

Nevertheless, all this info and Bad News can be used to create the Good News for you if or when he slips and starts nipping. That's because you now know in advance that he is almost sure to drink again! Indeed, there's nothing in the world you can do (short of weapons, of course) to prevent it.

The Good part of this News is that it means you no longer have to check on whether he has. It's only a matter of time, love, until it will be blatantly clear. In short order, you won't be able to miss it!

So relax. Just let him tell on himself. He most certainly will within a very short time of starting again.

Don't tense up another day of your life wondering if he's going to get drunk. It's like wondering if the sun is going to rise. That's because he's at least 90 percent sure to drink, and drink in the same old way that was causing trouble before.

Here's your trick: Set up some safety nets for yourself (and children), begin making whatever plans you need to in order to get peace for yourself, yet still get your basic needs met under the conditions that prevail when he's drinking.

Is that negative thinking? Is that looking for the worst? No! Most certainly not. It's not negative thinking to know that aftershocks follow earthquakes and prepare for them and protect yourself. It's not negative thinking to know that if a fire starts in your house you don't have to wait 'til the flames are a certain height to call the fire department.

Knowing this fact about problem drinking allows you to plan for the crashes, be ready for them, not be thrown for a loop by them. It allows you to quit worrying if he will mess up. He will. But knowing it in advance means you won't be shocked, or caught off guard, feel let down ,or hurt.

It is sane thinking to understand that after taking a drink, an over-drinker will very soon be taking another. Thinking otherwise is your problem thinking; it's believing a fantasy you wish were true.

Eight or more checkmarks on the changes list

Eight or more checkmarks guarantees that you are in significant emotional pain and have been for quite a while. What's more, eight or more checkmarks also means that his chances of really quitting are now even slimmer. That's because every time he drinks, the alcohol continues chopping away at his brain cells. By eight checkmarks, he will already have lost much of the mental capacity that is needed to quit and stay quit.

Surviving the rapid mood swings that come with living with an over-drinker, you will surely have tried to numb your awareness of how bad things have become. This response in you to what he's doing shows that you already have deep mental and emotional wounds.

None of you are wimps (no matter what you sometimes think). The real you, every one of you, is a fighter; you're spunky. Yet by now his behavior and repeated ugly comments will have cut deep marks into you. I call these emotional harms "wounds." Emotional scars are what's left when it quits bleeding and hurting so bad. These wounds and their scars will begin to alter your natural, beautiful personality. Worse, the scars and changes generally stay with the victim for their lifetime—unless they realize that it's rather easy, with qualified help, to mend your soul. You can heal and rebuild your assaulted spirit, your mind, your emotions. This book is your first step, and it's a giant step, toward precisely that—healing and rebuilding.

What Does the Checklist Score Suggest About Him?

_____

_____

And What Does Your Score Suggest About Your Situation?

_____

_____

Sure, Your Relationship Has

Some of the Same Problems that others have, *but* . . .
The first question I usually get at this point when I'm speaking or doing a workshop is usually about last chapter's list of how over-drinking affects a relationship. Your sisters say, "But don't all relationships get these same problems?"

Very astute of you if you want to ask that yourself. Your answer: "Sort of."

Some Important Differences
Healthy relationships do get some of those problems. But that is only a partial answer—and it's misleading. Although all relationships have problems—healthy people work on them successfully. They work together. In mutual respect and gentle patience. And they don't let problems sit, so they don't pile up. When healthy couples eventually resolve a problem, the solution pretty much equally satisfies both of them.

That's not the way it works in an over-drinker's relationship.

Love and intimacy are difficult to create and maintain even without a partner's over-drinking to complicate or cause them.

Let's look at some of the clear differences between healthy and unhealthy relationships, in terms of their problems:

1. In healthy relationships, both people equally work to resolve problems. One is not left to stew while the other drops out.

2. In healthy relationships, neither party gives in more than 50 percent of the time. And both stay carefully aware of this, out of care for one another.

3. In healthy relationships, problems don't pile up because the couple resolves them as they arise.

4. In healthy relationships, no one fears discussing a problem.

5. In healthy relationships, discussions about problems are respectful; each partner respecting and showing that respect for the other's feelings and intelligence.

6. In healthy relationships, each person accepts that all

people see things differently; therefore, they expect differences, and take time to understand each other's perspective, what the other thinks and why they think that, before making decisions.

7. In healthy relationships, both people's needs and desires are respected. All the time.

8. In healthy relationships no one is ever ridiculed or put down. Each assumes the other person is intelligent and means well.

9. In healthy relationships, issues are discussed in a trusting manner, knowing their partner will respect one's thinking.

10. In healthy relationships, no one fears the other will blow up over something the other one says. Both can relax.

11. In healthy relationships, no one ever calls the other names.

12. In healthy relationships, neither party brings up past errors or misdeeds. (A deliberate move to weaken the other person)

I list these necessary elements of a healthy relationship for those of you who don't really know how healthy relationships actually work. I've found that this is a good percentage of those I have worked with. If that is the case, it's not because you are bad; it's because you never learned how to do all these things. No one showed you, no one did them where you could watch and learn, no one modeled the healthy behaviors required to build a healthy relationship. People (and most animals) are wired to use their parents and other adults as their teachers, teaching them the way to conduct themselves.

You cannot know something you were never taught!

In addition, many of you haven't had the opportunity to observe a healthy relationship function. I know that because, if you had, you would not have settled for unhealthy behavior long before now. You—like the lucky girls who were taught these things—would have pulled up stakes long before you got in so deep. But you didn't know.

And to criticize yourself for not doing better is like beating yourself up for not being able to speak Chinese, or work out calculus problems. If no one has taught you that language, or that much math, not you and not anyone else, not even Einstein, could do it.

It's not because you are inferior or weak.

Another point is that you have the right to live in a partnership where the "rules" of a healthy relationship are sacred and followed, where they are always in effect. This is a great time to start working on that—whether you stay in this relationship or not. Reading over and over the facts about healthy relationships listed on pages 52 and 53, learning and practicing those rules you've not known about, even if your partner isn't willing. That's because you will never be able to have a healthy relationship, a relationship that meets your human needs, without also having these understandings in place.

(If nothing else, getting familiar with these rules is good practice for you for your next relationship—which is far more likely to be sooner than later if he isn't willing to work with you on learning these guidelines. A hidden benefit to beginning to study and think about these "rules" is that you'll recognize immediately if a new prospect doesn't use them. You'll never again get in so deep with a man "who has problems. You'll recognize and heed the early signs, knowing what they mean.

If your current partner isn't too far gone, share the list with him. Just don't expect a miracle. Most men who have become over-drinkers will ridicule both these rules and you. When that happens don't think it's because you did it wrong. It's not you!

All couples have differences that can cause problems. But what makes a relationships healthy or unhealthy is not whether they encounter problems; it's how they handle them. Sadly, you, on your own, cannot do it. Unless both of you learn the rules of a healthy relationship problem-solving, and work at using them, neither of you will ever have a healthy relationship. And unless you insist that any other prospective partners understand and use these guidelines, you're in for more of what you have now.

Another big difference in healthy relationships is that problems rarely pile up; rarely will either partner have to cope with several issues and pressures at once. Using the "rules" helps keep a clear slate and is proof against lingering arguments and problem pile-ups. Except in true catastrophe, partners in a healthy relationship never have a load of issues clogging up their brains at the same time. The result is that they are far less stressed, which means they are rarely snappish, impatient, distracted, worn down. What's more, neither of them will find themselves obsessing on a problem. They simply wait to have a healthy discussion and solution search with their true partner.

> **Psych Note:** Domestic violence is common in the homes of over-drinkers. Mixing alcohol (which dulls self-control) with the exaggerated rage response common in over-drinkers can be deadly. And he may not remember any of it.

More than 2,000 women each are killed by their intimate partners—many during such explosions. Those 2,000 a year are only the dead women whose partners are finally convicted of killing them; that's why we suspect at least double this number is reality. And those are only the ones caught and then found guilty. All doubtful murders are not on the final reports at this time. All this tells you that the average number of women killed by the man closest to them is at least 40 women every year per state: In your state. Do not be number 41. And he may not remember any of it. Go immediately to Chapter 9 for more info if this fits you. Then you can come back here and continue. The information in Chapter 9 is so important to the woman whose drinker can also get mean that you never read anything else in your life, you must read Chapter 9.

Many of you can learn a few tricks and live more comfortably (I'm not saying "nicely.") with your over-drinker. **If, however, he has ever become violent, or if you've begun to fear that he may become violent, there are no safe fixes.**

You now must begin to trust your instincts fully. You've likely come to doubt yourself, your judgement, but here's the trick to cure that:

The Trust-Your-Instincts Trick

1. You start with Catch It! The moment you begin to sense he even possibly may become violent.

2. Immediately Think: "If I Move Along now, I may look like a fool, make him more angry. But if I'm right, and I Move Along, I keep my face unscarred, myself from being injured—physically or emotionally!"

(Note: If even the hint of violence is any part of your case,

go immediately to Chapter 9. Read and take to heart the information, then act on it. You can come back and the rest of this chapter later.)

> **Psych Note:** If it's safe, and you choose to stay with your man, one tactic can bring some healing to your relationship:
>
> **When you are angry at him,
> curse the behavior, not the man.**

"I hate your bad temper!" not "I hate you!"
"I hate the things you are doing," rather than "I hate you."

An over-drinker's mind is impaired—even when he's not drinking. Many of his thinking cells are damaged. Or gone.

As a result, a man who has never been violent can become so, because especially impaired is his judgement, and his ability to maintain control of his emotions, as well as his behavior. (You will see this in his bursts of anger, his rage (intense, physically expressed anger). Many of you see it in his jealousy, and in his over-sensitive ego. Whether or not you've seen any sign of potential violence, you must determine now to always trust your intuition in questions of safety.

If you get a hint there may be violence, don't even take the time to question or calm the situation; gently shut down discussion and find a way to leave the area. (Remember: No one can guarantee your safety with a man who over-drinks. So many women who are dead now once said, "but I know he's never really hurt me.")

Don't worry about hurting his pride or making him more angry. Indeed, if those reactions are possible, it reinforces the fact that you may be living with a violent man. If that man is not physically violent yet, he has already inflicted harmful emotional violence on you. We know this is true, or you would not fear upsetting him.

Your number one prerogative right now must start being yourself—your welfare, not his ego, not his feelings; he's passed beyond the point where your caring is enough to squelch his drive. His ego or hurt feelings are a minor loss compared to you or your children being crippled in a wreck. Safety is always your priority, not his hurt feelings. You live with a man whose judgement and behavior control is crashing. Even one who has never been violent in the past can lose control—without warning.

Let's get to the Stars in your new Bag of Tricks!

The Stretchy-Lip Trick and The Move Along Trick

Let's start working on your first two new tricks. They're simple. Each of them are tricks in their own right, usable at almost any time and easily done as a team or separately to great effect. Both also are part of most other tricks in this book. Either trick as a stand-alone can create an opening to escape ugly or tense moments. They are still more valuable, easy as they are, because you can pull either or both out long before a situation gets tense, thus saving you the usual stress.

I call the first trick "The Stretchy-Lip Smile," and the second, "Move Along!" Both are as simple as their names suggest, with only a few easy steps. (Having only a few steps to remember is a huge plus when there's tension because tension freezes the brain, blocks clear thinking and thoughtful responding.

(The Stretchy-Lip Trick. Imagine! You, the Queen of the Smiley Face, are going to get a lesson in smiling. It's okay to chuckle here.)

Studying this smile is not because you don't know how to smile! It's because you don't know how to smile when it will make all the difference. *When it will create surprise.* And you use it when you won't feel like smiling.

You will learn and practice these easy tricks a few times so they are as comfortable as old slippers and flow from you as naturally as the prettiest river you've ever seen. Practice, if only by thinking about their steps, keeps them oiled and cleaned, ready for a quick draw.

Point to Remember: Your stretchy-lip smile trick will never be triggered by happiness; it will always be triggered only by tension. When you feel or even anticipate tension, that's the signal for these tricks to slide on-stage.

Few people naturally react to stress with a smile, but it's easier to make it a habit than you may think. All that's needed is using a trick and seeing it work to engrave it in permanent ink. You quickly become graceful, natural in using these tricks because they are so effective; they bring such a good reward that both your conscious and subconscious mind pounce on them and paste them in, prodding you, reminding you to use them.

You'll soon attend to your body's responses—tension—to recognize stress. Your body tells you when you're thirsty or hungry and it tells you when you are tense. Some of the warnings are jumpiness, too quick reflexes, tight shoulders, clenched jaw, stiff neck. When you sense pressure building you know it's time to pull out your tricks, and get a break to ponder what's going on.

The idea of keeping tabs on their own stress level can be daunting, but let me remind you—you are already a master of this skill—that is, sensing rising stress in others. Especially him. What tells you someone else is getting pressured? Whatever you see or feel, use the same senses to detect your own stress. You don't have to wait until your stress reaches a certain level before using a trick. Use a trick as soon as you notice any of your signs. The sooner, the better. Stretchy Lip, Move Along.

An Add-on to Most Tricks

You'll often be reminded to loosen up after most tricks. This is the "Now, go do something fun" step. Your goal is to pull out this trick for coming down off tension. Also as a reward for the Very Good Girl inside you. **Go do something fun.**

Something Fun?

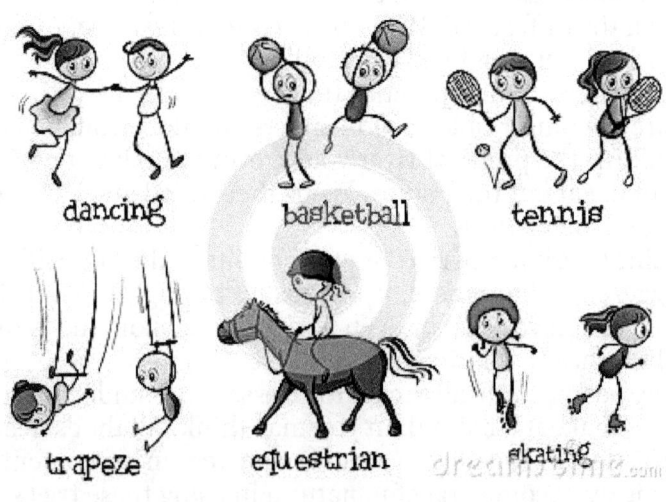

dancing   basketball   tennis

trapeze   equestrian   skating

* * *

Stretchy-Lip and Move Along produce a great side-effect:

They strengthen your sense of dignity.

This element is important; a part of you has cringed and felt like a wimp emotional explosions or just crumpling to whatever is being demanded.

Learning these tricks isn't just for dealing with him; when *anyone* begins to criticize you or complain about what you do or how you do it, these tricks are properly used then too. And they work.

The other party may stay riled up, but you are creating for yourself a graceful way to avoid being hit with the rotten apples others can throw.

Here's the secret power of these tricks: *The Surprise.*

A surprise, even a tiny one, creates a brief Brain Freeze. Surprise is what happens when you expect one thing, but get something unexpected. Surprise!

The surprise coming from these tricks is because he's expecting you to do what you usually do when he begins his stuff.

This time he's going to get something different. Surprise!

His Brain Freeze, no matter how small, allows you to make an exit.

Surprise! It creates potent brain chemicals (Fight or Flight body chemistry that we'll discuss later). That stall out the mind I call Brain Freeze, and Bambi Brain. The stall lasts from a few seconds to several minutes, and its always possible brevity is why you immediately follow up your surprise smile with its mate, surprise Move Along.

Surprise: Think about what your usual response is when he starts being nasty, or criticizing you. What is your usual response? . (Do you puff up and pop off at him in return? Or do you crumple and feel like a total loser? Do you fly back at him with reminders of his own imperfections? Do you argue with whatever he says, trying to defend yourself or show him that he's wrong? All of the above? And have any of those ever set things right nicely? No?

Know that whatever your usual response is, that's what he's expecting now. But from now on, as soon as you catch it, you're going to do something a little different.

He has just done the usual thing, and he expects you to do your usual thing. And that is what sets up the surprise, an event that briefly stuns him and gives you a second or two to Move Along, Stretchy-Lip pasted on.

Why Does He Do the Things He Does?

When he starts most of his stuff, he doesn't really care if he's wrong. He's just producing something he has learned fills his need to let off steam; he'll fire it at whoever is close—or whoever he believes will let him get away with it. (He uses all of his tricks because he knows they will produce the response he wants you to produce. And how does he know? Aha! You've taught him. He says "a" and you shout "b". He knows exactly which of his words will trigger in you the response he's trying to get from you.

No matter how you try to defend yourself when he makes his sarcastic or just plain wrong statements or accusations; your defenses will never work. He actually uses them to pump up the tension, in hopes of getting you to break.

You see, it's almost never about whatever he says it is. It's all about whatever he's trying to make happen, a manipulation. That's why he always finds a way around whatever you say to defend yourself with another criticism of you, or he just blows you off (disrespectfully).

Truth is not his objective; blowing off steam or getting you into a bad situation are.

Additionally, he only uses a trick where he believes he can get away with it. Either because you'll crumple, or because no one else is present. Most often, he wants to get your goat. Why would he deliberately upset you? That's his way to get something else he's after.

Once he provokes you into a corner, he'll likely say, "See, you've done it again! I'm out of here!"

Slam!

Why would he want to get your goat? Upset you deliberately? Because he hates you? Nope.

It's because when he gets your goat he instantly takes control—of the situation, and of you.

The whole thing was about his needing to either dump on you, verbally demote you so he can feel superior—his security blanket (picture him sucking his thumb and holding his security blanket). Or he uses this technique to gain control after you crack. Actually, he has total control once you come back at him with the first thing he says or does.

You'll never win doing what you've always done. Well, have you? That's because you are responding rationally to the irrational set-up he creates.

Answering any of his comments or responding to something

he does is what he's looking for. Not only is it breaking you down, it's making him the King.

Any answer you make to one of his critical or snide remarks can only hurt you. That's because, when you respond, you aim for what he's said, and that's the wrong target. Shooting at the wrong target you score zero.

Your options: Throw up your hands in early surrender, "You win!" or figure out what he's after and let him have it as you Move Along (on your way to do something fun--a brief break for you, a reward for your Inner Actress and your Inner Child.

When you dispute what he says, you won't win. Figure what he wants, give it to him if you can, but for sure Move Along.

Otherwise, you'll get and stay mad, very hard on your mental and emotional condition. Certainly, you can lose the better part of the day to it.

Behind all of his antics are his subconscious reasons: No matter what he words say about you, it's just not about you.

He's creating an opening to leave the house to get a drink, and drink the way he wants to—and then he can blame it on you because you just blew up or said so-and-so.

He now leaves to go without guilt (Slam!) if he convinces you that he's leaving because you are so awful. He leaves in great good humor.

Just remember: He will go to great lengths to get you do or say something he can point to, saying, "It's all your fault!" Watch and see next time.

He consciously and subconsciously does what he's doing to create specific responses in you. And he knows just how to get there. How does he know what to do? Why--you've taught him! Not intentionally, but every time you come back at him, he knows he's stirred you up, and he knows what to do next time. When you remember that his subconscious wants to make him feel powerful (because he doesn't) and in control of something. His subconscious also aids and abets letting him get out and drink freely, and it's a bonus when he can blame it all on you.

Slam!

But this time can be different: He does his thing. You give him Stretchy-Lip. Brief brain stall, Brain Freeze—like when you eat ice cream too fast. Then he'll repeat whatever usually works, but by now you are into your Move Along strut.

The surprise effect usually lasts long enough for you to gracefully Move Along. Strive be graceful, to keep from energizing him, but even at worst, getting away is away. Go for it!

His initial Brain Freeze will be followed by mental work, trying to figure out what's going on with you. He will go do what he wanted to do, but he won't be feeling joyous, or powerful.

The goal of your Move Along is to get out of ear-shot, first to cut your chances of wanting to say something back (Do not! Pinch your lips together like holding a mouse by the tail!) Move Along.

Go somewhere pleasant and there, take a short break to plan your next step toward your current favorite project or goal.

If you are stirred up, take a brisk walk.

More About "Brain Freeze"

You know how, when someone jumps out at you and you startle? And after that you don't function well for a while? This is what you create in your mate with the Stretchy Lip Smile when he's expecting something quite different—a comeback. Surprise pumps out chemicals that freeze the body and brain briefly as it prepares to Fight or Escape. Arguing with what he says only fires him up higher. Your job is to Stretch those lips, Camp those jaws, and Move Along

Making new responses doesn't come any easier than learning to ride a bike came easy. But like riding the bike, or saying your ABCs, all you need is to do it over and over. Just thinking about a trick is practice. As you practice, look at yourself in the mirror; practice the new trick it while imagining him going into an uproar. See yourself calmly Stretch 'Em, and Moving Along. Mentally take the time to pat yourself on the back each time.

While pulling your Stretchy-Lip Smile is simple, the hard part is the timing: H initial "stuff," whatever he uses to get your goat, can create Brain Freeze in you. That's why you practice, the more often, the less likely is Brain Freeze. You'll be ready. Strive toward thinking through and practicing several times a day each of your new tricks. The result will be that, even if you freeze up mentally, your body will reflexively do what you've been training it to do.

Here's a promise: Once you begin using these tricks, they

rapidly sink in and begin to flow naturally. Know why? Because they work so well. Your subconscious perceives success as a reward.

Dead-stopping a habitual response is difficult, if not impossible; few have the ability to do that. But replacing one reflex with a new one has been proved successful over and over. Indeed, it's your answer to "How to change myself?"

In this case, when you are feeling tense, getting fired up, go directly for Stretching your Lips. With practice your subconscious mind takes over, as surely as a tennis star almost unconsciously slams that backhand.

> **Psych Note:** Once a new way of responding succeeds in getting what you want—in this case, getting out of range and finding something nice to do—that new response rapidly becomes your new (and more successful) way of responding to the same prod.

You're going to enjoy your new tricks because of their effect on him: You might say they are "stunning." You begin to see that you have the power to stop him in his tracks. That means, you take control of the situation as to how much misery you're going to suffer. What you need now is a handful of opportunities to practice the new ways.

Oh—but you have that! He's still him. He'll be giving you many opportunities to practice, and you're going to get really good.

This means you cease dreading his getting ugly, being a butt; now you hope he will so you get another chance to practice!

How do star golfers learn their spectacular techniques? Concert musicians? Star footballers? Tennis stars? Piano masters? Right. They use this same technique: mentally visualizing themselves doing the new thing successfully and feeling it and being happy about it. This simple technique works for the great professionals and it will work for you.

> **CAUTION—DANGER!—CAUTION**
>
> **DO NOT use any of these tricks on a violent man!**

> **If a Man has Ever Been Violent, Go to Chapter 9. First read it, then return here. You need that information as soon as you can get it.**

> **DO NOT disagree with this man once you sense he's moving toward a mean state.**
> You do this, not to let him win, but to spare yourself grief. Possibly danger.
> Besides, you've probably tried before, but it doesn't work, does it?
> Has it ever?

At this point, you can have some fun: Draw on your little Inner Actress, you know, the one that is perfectly capable of saying, "Whatever you say, dear," or "Oh, I'm just fine!" "Yes, Honey."

Then Move Along to whatever you intended before all this blew up, or just Move Along to go do something fun. Away from where he can easily be heard to halt the temptation to answer him back.

Go do something fun for a while.

What's fun? Some ideas!

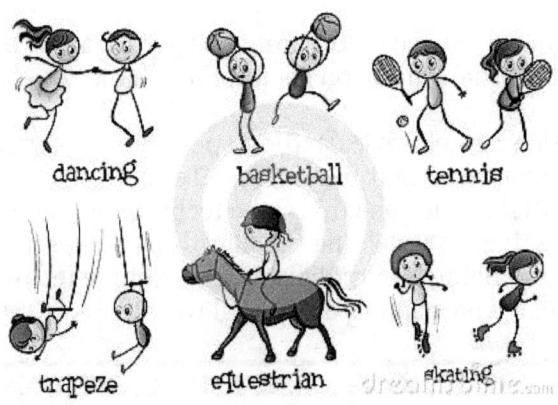

Moving Right Along

Never, ever squat while wearing spurs!
And never, ever argue with a man who can become violent.

What does it matter if you win your point but get a broken jaw? You've already seen that even when you win a point, it rarely does any good.

Engrave this in your mind: No argument can change his attitude, except by making it worse--no matter how right you are!

His rage creates a form of Brain Freeze. His intelligent brain (what's left of it) is temporarily frozen, so he will not, cannot, "get" your point. And he certainly won't adjust his attitude at the drop of a bright comment. The terrible possibility is that you can get hurt. All those things are just too much to pay simply to get a word in—a word that has never had the effect you want.

In fact, saying anything except some form of "Yes Honey," at these times, is sure to fire him up worse. The biggest part of him *wants* you to come back at him, that part of him that is looking to dump all his tensed-up and uncomfortable feelings.

Yes, I know answering his sarcasm or criticism or whatever is a knee-jerk reaction; I've been there. But I, like so many others, have found that the Smile and Move Along are skills that anyone can learn, and quickly.

You burst out and argue with whatever he has said because he's just dead wrong—but now you can see that any resistance, or argument, is a trigger for the man wanting to dump his tense, rageful feelings.

Arguing or resisting don't calm him; they fire up his energy, they build his rage. Then, because he lacks adequate controls, the rage he's probably carried with him since childhood totally swamps his brain which then takes over because of his diminished ability to control himself.

He can be like a bursting dam under the power of brain and body chemicals demand action.

Unexpected submission will usually throw a wrench into anyone's exploding rage gears. It is a small surprise. It can slow him. Do not use a surprise he can take as threatening. You can only surprise this man with something utterly non-threatening. Mild surprise is your goal. Move Along, without Stretchy Lip in tense situations. It can be taken as you being nasty.

Yes, you have the right to resist, but resistance with a man who drinks too much is not only dangerous, but practically guaranteed to be useless!

Put your own drives aside for now; focus on finding the best path away.

Few points are worth creating the kind of risk involved here in coming back at him with resistance. A man who has never been violent can become so; a man who has already been violent can become more so.

Always Take The Safe Route! Small dishonesties can be forgiven. Issues can be addressed later.

* * *

> **Psych Note:** None of the tricks in this book can be certified as safe for use with a man who has any tendency to become violent.
>
> If violence is even a remote possibly, you begin to realize the danger to a woman when alcohol, which relaxes the behavior control part of his brain, is mixed in. Even small amounts.
>
> Of women killed by their partners, a large number believed, and even told others, "He won't really hurt me." They didn't think he would. But the alcohol-affected brain just isn't the man you think you know.
>
> **You cannot safely use any trick at all with a man who has any tendency to violence, which includes any man who has even threatened it, or mentioned it. What you must do is Go Now to Chapter 9; use the information there before reading any further here.**
>
> You can never be sure of safety around a violent man, drinking or not. The man who simply threatens violence is already capable of acting on it.
>
> Add alcohol, which lowers inhibitions and his behavior control, and you are standing in front of a time bomb.
>
> How do I know these things? I have made research and work in this field of psychology a major focus for over 40 years. And I lived it myself. For many years. With not one, but two such partners.
>
> Even if he's not violent now, as he continues to disintegrate

> he may well become so.

In the past 40 years, I've read and studied hundreds of cases, hundreds of reports, detailing cases of violence on women. I've read hundreds of death notices of women killed by their partners. That's how I know all this and why I take it very seriously, why I am determined to get these messages out you.

Your new these tricks will come quickly to you, but it will be a very long time before they are not the surprise of his day.

Now we go in-depth with the Stretchy-Lip Smile Trick. It has only three simple steps, but, as it is our first trick, I include a lot of psychological commentary to give you a stronger sense of how and why the trick works so well.

No trick can be sure of working every time: An Olympic ice-skater sometimes falls down; a golf pro and a star field-goal kicker sometimes miss their shot. This only reminds you that you need to add a few easy tricks to ride along with these first few. Mentally practicing your new ways of responding will strengthen your ability to do them when you need them. You will soon be amazed, both at yourself and the difference it makes with him.

While you will rarely do these things perfectly, you can almost always work out pieces of them, and even small pieces of these tricks can still get an effect.

The Good News is that, if you mess up any part of a trick, just keep on (if it's reasonable and safe); rely on other parts of the trick to do their job.

The Stretchy-Lip Smile Trick

Step 1. Catch it! You learn to recognize your time of need. Catch the moment. (It's when you either want to scream or smack him.)

You quickly learn to be sensitive to rising tension. Rising tension is the blast that you now use to fire off the Stretchy-Lip Smile. Don't wait to get more tense once you sense any; go ahead and act then. There are rarely any errors, although most seem to fear acting too soon. But so what if you do? So what if you leave a situation before both of you are worked up too high?

You can't control his emotions or outbursts, but you can always spot them. Now begin to respond immediately—Stretch Lips, Move Feet.

> **Psych Note:** It's virtually impossible to stop an emotional

explosion once it begins. This is why we work on the part that's much easier to control—the build-up to the bang.

Trying to stop yourself (or him) once the explosion occurs is hopeless. You're trying to stop all the air from leaving the balloon when it bursts.

No, you have to go about this differently—catch it! Catch it before the boom. Built-up emotions are like water balloons. When the pressure of added water reaches their maximum capacity. they explode. Your inner balloon was never created to hold so much frustration and pain, and the inescapable stress that comes with a progressing over-drinker. Consequently, it's just a matter of time until it blows. Until you blow. It's not a catastrophe! It's the natural result that points out what you've been doing wrong. Bang!

When a too-full balloon bursts, it doesn't mean the balloon is flawed. Cut yourself some slack, girl. The problem isn't that you explode; that's the natural way of things. Your problem is how much is being stuffed into your balloon just so you can function.

The first step to learning a new way is this: Learn to Catch It! You do that by thinking how it feels when you're reaching your last ragged rope. Think about how your body reacts just thinking about it.

Your uncomfortable reactions are going to become your early warning system. The coming tricks make it possible for you to slip like an eel out of a tight spot.

Tension starts when your brain interprets what you hear, see, smell, or feel has any kind of threat to it. In nanoseconds this nearly subconscious part of you can pick this up.

To help you spot tension, think of it as a balloon. Tension is produced from both body and brain chemicals whose purpose is to prepare you for a possible emergency, preparing you to either escape or giving extra strength to defend yourself: Fight or Flight. Those chemicals begin filling your balloon. It increases, grows, so long as any part of you believes something may be a threat. His tension works the same way. The difference is that he is more sensitive to threat than you are.

Your balloons keep filling up, increased tension creating powerful energy-. When your emotional balloon pops, you can't stop it—no more than you can stop a real balloon once it begins to pop.

This is why you are learning a way to catch it before it reaches its max. Your max depends on many things: how well you slept last night, what else has been going on and stressing you, if you've been eating right, if you're healthy or not, and on and on.

You need a way not only to catch your tension building, but to catch it before it goes too far—and since you can't be sure how far is too far at a given time, you must learn to stop it as soon as you become aware of it.

Then you Stretchy-Lip him and Move Along.

Tension is easy to spot because it's uncomfortable, and that's Good News. The discomfort tension creates makes it easier to spot early and use a trick to prevent your popping. The quicker you spot tension rising and Move Along, the sooner it settles down. Here's a clue to picking up on your tension the first few dozen times:

It's when you feel the urge to leap over the table to grab or smack him. Catch it then! It's almost too late!

Immediately turn your focus to clamping your jaws and lips and stretching 'em.

(Note: Other women have reported that while choking, shooting, and pan-slamming him may stop what their partner is doing, it's only temporary. Worse, your kind of sweet spirited women feel terrible, and guilty for doing those things. So whopping him turns out to bring little satisfaction. Well—some say it brings satisfaction, but it doesn't last long after the police arrive.)

* * *

Step 2. Clamp 'Em. Tightly Clamp your jaws and lips! (Breathe normally while clamped!) Clamping your jaws together and sealing your lips produce at least these four splendid results:

1) Clamped jaws and lips can't say anything back to him, can't defend, can't argue, can't throw more gasoline on his fire.

2) Not saying anything back, you can't get hooked into his attempt to manipulate you. Remember, he knows, if only subconsciously, that if he gets you upset, he can take control of the situation.

(Note: You tend to labor under the mistaken belief that something you say is really going to change his mind.)

3) The third benefit of the Stretchy-Lip Smile: It forces your focus off whatever he's saying—if only briefly. But briefly is all

that's needed to pause the burst of chemicals in your body and avoid being wounded by anything he says. You slow your balloon's filling.

4) The fourth benefit of Stretchy-Lip: Relief from tension. Tension leaving the body feels really good! (And that is the payoff tha triggers your subconscious to get on board with this trick.)

Step 3. Stretch 'Em! With jaws and lips tightly clamped, stretch the corners of your mouth back toward your ears. Voila! It's Magic! To others, this stretching looks like a smile! Not only is this expression usually a surprise (which interrupts most tirades), it's also extremely hard-to-read. (Think Mona Lisa.)

Okay, here's your Condensed Version, the only one you need once you understand the explanations of how the trick works and why.

Step 1. Catch It!
Step 2. Clamp 'Em!
Step 3. Stretch 'Em!

* * *

Psych Note: Confusion and brain-stall are the universal responses to surprise—even in animals. With Stretchy-Lip, you are using a nonthreatening surprise to swerve away from a head-on collision. (And then there's that sensation of joy when you see his face change, as he tries to figure you out.

One of the great things about Stretchy-Lip is that although using it immediately—as soon as tension rises—is best, it still has a powerful impact at any point you remember to do it

**Practice makes Progress, not Perfection.
(Making Progress is Enough!)**

**Always Celebrate the Tiniest Bit of Progress!
Make a Big Deal of it in your own head.
Indeed—It IS a Big Deal!**

Talk about surprise effects: Much of the effect his bad

behavior has had on you has come from the surprise of certain things he says and does. And when he blows up, often you aren't expecting it--surprise. When his blowups surprise you, it's you going into Brain Freeze. (You may later ask yourself, "Why didn't I say this or that?" Now you know.)

* * *

A New Reflex Reaction to His "Stuff"

Occasionally practice your Stretchy-Lip Smile in front of a mirror. Check your look: You don't want to appear to snarl, or look like you're having cramps. Work on it until you master the look you want to put forth. (Hold your head high; this gives an impression of grace and calm—even if you don't have either.)

This is another place where Bad News can be flipped into Good News. The Bad News, that he's probably never going to change much, turns into Good News because his same-old self is going to give you ample opportunities to practice your new Smile. (What makes a new trick become like a reflex, crowding other reflexes out, is simple: It's just practice, repetition.

Practicing is easy. Do it during your time alone (lest you be misunderstood—or reported to the authorities). But most of you get to be alone frequently. When you drive around doing boring chores, are stuck in traffic, when you cook, scrub, do dishes, clean up messes, clean the bathroom. You're alone. And waiting for him to come home.

Now you can use all your alone time to start practicing each new trick. Practice it, get the words right, your voice right, your facial expression right. It takes practice. Over and over. How many times does that beautiful skater practice her graceful turns? You practice a new trick that many times.

But you'll be quite good at all of them long before then. They really are easy; it's just learning them. And they work so well that one you apply one, part of you can't wait to do it again.

Once you use Stretchy-Lip, he's hooked. He can't figure you out; most men hate that. They're wired that way (likely for survival of the race). He needs to figure things out and when he can't, it begins to eat on him. And that's when it gets a lot of attention. This means that you're going to be on his mind a lot once you start using these tricks! In fact, you are well on your way to becoming the Mystery Woman in his life.

DO NOT, NEVER EVER, explain to him what you're doing!

When he figures it out, it quits working (as well).

Keep your secret and the trick keeps on working.

> **Psych Note:** When you are stressed or upset, your body produces chemicals that prime it to fight or run away. Intense stress can cause freezing (think Bambi in the headlights). That makes it an excellent tool for your purposes—putting space between you and an argumentative person.

If you don't begin to move when stressed, the flooding chemistry of stress causes you to become uncomfortable, agitated, irritable—all of which is a set-up for an explosion

The simple trick, Move Along, gives you complete control of your own life and behavior in those times.

Walking is a great stress reducer; brisk walking even better. Both burn up those fiery biochemicals that give you those unpleasant feelings (antsy) when you become anxious or stressed. So get moving! And pick up the pace!

Trying to reduce your stress or anxiety by trying to calm down will not work, cannot work. The mandates of polite society are dead wrong on this point. Sitting still is not a stress reducer. It's impossible to relax with stress chemicals flooding your body.

Just Move Along until you feel relief from tension, feel your brain slow down. Should you feel tension creeping back in, pick up your pace again. To the best of your ability at the moment though, don't Move Along fast until you are clear of him. A swift movement on your part could set him off if he's in a temper; it also signals that you are upset—which is just what he wants.

Once you're clear of him, Move Along as fast as you please. If you're a jogger, or a bike rider or skater or whatever—do it! Your medicine now, your calm-down pill is action. The icing is for you to head for do something fun, even if you can only spare moments. (Often, just the thought of something you'd like to be doing is enough to stir up those happy chemicals that diminish and negate the irritable, antsy chemicals of stress.

The stress-anxiety chemicals (in addition to making you uncomfortable) can harm you. Not only do they trigger you to do or say all the things that have never worked before, those chemicals—which were never meant to be long-term in your system—begin to damage your body. (Think stomach upset, a crick in the neck, a headache—consequences of organs being hammered by these biochemicals.

One thing for sure: There's no way you can regret what you say if your jaws and lips are locked.

* * *

Your Next New Trick

For now—and at least until you complete this book—put off saying anything at all to him about his drinking or behavior—as best you can. You already know that if you say anything—anything!—about his drinking, he'll puff up and become hostile. (And now you will start expecting him to react that way, so you won't be surprised, because surprise interferes with logical thought.) No matter how many times he has promised to behave, you must keep a part of your mind ready for the most likely outcome: repeat behaviors.

Now you also know that his most used trick—emotional intimidation, which even if unspoken still means "If you don't stop what you're doing, I'm going to get real ugly." (Sheesh—only someone who is already real ugly would use such a threat!)

The over-drinker is invested in shutting out negative comments about his drinking, thus your attempts to enlighten him cannot succeed. So I ask you: Why bother? (Has it worked so far?)

> **Psych Note:** Oddly, research shows that every time you argue about a point, each party is forced to defend their view, and that reinforces the strength of a mistaken belief. Psychology proves that arguing is not only useless, it's harmful. To you.

The over-drinker is world-class at shutting out or arguing down your comments, and his responses are aimed to hurt you because he knows that will shut you down. (Hint: Don't use your hurt as a tactic to get him to care; it never works past the first months of the relationship. Shut out the words by recalling that he has an impaired brain and whatever he says is bent.)

Yet even his arguing that his drinking isn't a problem isn't all Bad. In fact, it's Good. If he argues to defend his drinking, it proves that part of him knows he has come to need to drink. The thought of not having it now appears to his subconscious as a threat!

From this you learn that his problem is already far beyond the point where an intelligent argument will work on him. Back off and reassess: Is arguing anything with him worth what it does to you? No, because you don't ever really win.

Once you've told him anything about his drinking and behavior, however, it's in his head forever. Want proof? How often does he throw up to you something you have said to him in the past about his drinking? Anything he doesn't like, just as anything you've already said about his drinking? It's "in." He can't get rid of it.

> **The following trick takes advantage of the quirk we've just discussed:**
>
> Not saying anything about his drinking for a while sets him up for a very powerful trick. After a silence, the first thing hears gets in! He deeply hears i. You'll know it got in when he jumps back at you with "You said you weren't going to say anything!"
>
> You do not need to apologize. Let the force of h is words be all that's in the air as you leave him to think about it.

A Whole New Way of Seeing the World

What used to feel like Bad News—when he jumped right back at you when you said something—is actually Good News! When he does that, his knee-jerk proves that whatever you just said really, really got in!

Now--Just Stretch 'Em, Clamp 'Em, and Move Along.

> **Psych Note:** Now his jumping back at something you say tells you that you've hit a hot spot. And that's really Good News because his hot spots are connected to protecting his ego and his ability to drink the way he wants to. It's also like lowering the shields on the Starship Enterprise—his cocky way falls and up pops his wounded ego and his attempt to put you down is only a way he uses to be sure he gets to drink what and when he wants to. So next time he pops back at you, don't cringe—pat yourself on the back!
>
> Seeing his shouting for what it can diminish its power on you. You know he'll remember it. How? Think how many times he has

> thrown up something you said years ago just to get you going now? Oh, no, it gets in. He remembers every little thing he doesn't like. Take it to the bank.

This tactic is well worth the patience with yourself it will take to perfect it. Holding your tongue gets easier once you begin to see how powerful this little trick can be.

There's another benefit to holding back from saying anything for a while: If you say nothing at all about his drinking for a period, you get in return a space of time nearly free from fiery arguments.

* * *

The Save Your Comments Trick

Save up your comments when you want to say something to really smash through his hard head. Think of it this way: The less *said* now, the better he *hears* later.

Make notes of the things you are putting off saying so you can remember them once the tension starts rising.

* * *

The Quiet Time Trick

1. Tell him you're not going to say anything else about his drinking (and don't get dragged into discussing it: Simple answer like "I just don't want to talk about it any more," or the like.

2. Now Clamp 'em and Move Along). He won't take you seriously and you don't need to get into a conversation of this nature anyway.

3. When you want to scream about the drinking or whatever else he has done, Stop! Move Along, Escape! Remember that being quiet is setting him up! You are setting him up for a Triple Play—playing a Good Trick on him that can end up being as helpful to him as to you.

4. Remind yourself of the big reward you'll collect from using these tactics: It's that he'll actually hear you! The longer you put off saying it, the more power builds up behind it when said.

5. Now—Clamp 'Em and Move Along. (Your words will

eventually get said—and by holding it now, they'll later have an effect, whereas they won't now.)

(Note: Savor the reward of silence and peace from using this trick. It makes the whole trick easier to do. It only takes a time or two of savoring to grab your subconscious and it happily begins to help you when needed. And be patient with yourself. Fussing at yourself smothers the good feelings that come from this trick.)

Just getting in a word or two rarely accomplishes what you're after so why start World War III with a comment? Save it to use when it will count.

* * *

Mastering the Move Along Trick

This trick opens up space to make quick, easy escapes. It has only four steps, and works before an explosion occurs—when you just catch the tension building. Surprisingly, it also works during an explosion, but then you try to wait until he's finished *speaking* and drop the smile. This trick works even after the explosion. At all three times, it is surprising for him, and relief for you. Can't get much better than these four simple steps!

The Move-Along Trick

1. While your Stretchy-Lip Smile is jamming his gears, you force your focus on only moving one foot forward, pointing away from the problem, and toward an exit.

2. Next, deliberately lower your shoulders (so you appear relaxed even if you aren't).

3. Lean forward onto the foot pointing to an exit. This forces sliding the other foot forward. Repeat.

4. Keep on until you're not only out of sight and hearing, but until you feel yourself beginning to relax. (If you stop too soon, it's much too tempting for him to catch up to say something else mean.) Focus on moving your feet—and closing your ears. Move until you are out of his area. Then find a pleasant place to

regather yourself.

Add-On Trick to Move-Along:

The Talking to the Air Trick

1. As you begin to Move Along, place your hand lightly to your cheek.
2. Now say one of the following things (or something better that you make up):
   - **"Oh! do I smell smoke?"**
   - **"Oh! I left the stove on!"**
   - **"Oh! Was that the phone? (or door)"**
     and the all-time winner:
   "Oh! I need to go to the bathroom!"

Another Plug-In for Move Along
(Just one simple step.)

1. Often as you wish, think of your Inner Actress and release her as you begin Move Along.
Let her out.
She'll be thrilled to assist you.

Give your Move Along as much flair as you wish—swing your hips, do a beautiful, graceful Indian dances with your hands as you move away, yodel, shake your booty, surprise and distract. And that's all it takes to throw water on his fire. Temporarily, of course. A minor Brain Freeze does the job.

Questions of Great Import to Ponder

1. Just how trustworthy is his judgement of you? Especially when he is upset. Is it sane, are his judgements sound, correct?

_____

2. Whose brain is being eaten away so that he can't even manage himself? Is the brain that's left trustworthy?

_____

3. Has working for his approval (as a substitute for love)

brought you what you're really after? (Try respect, love.)

___

4. If you finally do please him, how long does it last?

___

Notes on this Chapter

When his words grab your focus, he wins—at least in his own mind. Certainly you lose something. It's not a total bust if you get hooked again; just as soon as you realize it, slam on Stretchy Lip and point that foot away in a solid Move Along.

Fringe benefit: At almost any point you remember to use them, these two tricks still work. Surprise and absence.

Let him stand there shouting or spouting off as you Move Along with your focus elsewhere. The new goal you run for is the payoff—that when he's spent, he caves, gets quieter. Not happier. Just quieter. Usually you hear a loud "Slam!"

If you're lucky, maybe he'll pout for a few days.

Perhaps the strongest Deep Trick is imprinting the reality that all of his tricks aim at one thing: Getting gratification, either to his ego, or for getting the feeling he wants via a drink. Also recall that he is not opposed to upsetting you to manipulate a situation. He has learned (even if only subconsciously) that when you are upset, he can easily take control.

Forcing your focus off him and onto clamping your jaws and moving your feet is like throwing up a cloak of invisibility over your ears. If you refuse to focus on whatever he's saying, those words just drift off into the air.

You Can Create Opportunities for Fun

I have observed that most drinkers's women have a robust Inner Actress. It's part of how they survive. She's probably always been there, and now I can confidently guarantee that she will be able to carry off all these tricks—with flair and more than a dab of fun at times.

Just pull her out once; you and your subconscious will be hooked. She'll begin to pop up whenever she's needed.

> *Special Note to the woman with a difficult man: The experience of a sizeable number of women has been that firearms and other weapons do not enhance the techniques you'll learn here. It is our—I mean, their experience that, while weapons may let you get the upper hand, your success is brief. It stops as soon as you put the gun or whip down to take care of the kids. Or you fall asleep. Or go to the bathroom. Even worse, he can file felony charges! Jails are so ugly nowadays that, even though it can give you a delicious break from the grind, it's not your best option. For all the above reasons, shun weapons.*

Let's rehearse the main tricks from this chapter. What does repetition do? Right! Makes things more readily accessible, even when you're under stress. The more practice, the easier the new thing will come.

I. Stretchy-Lip Smile—with Move-Along

1. Catch the moment (you feel tension building)!

2. Clamp those jaws!

3. Stretch those lips!

4. Put out one foot in the direction of "away," then lean on it.

5. Now slide the other foot forward and repeat Steps 4 and 5.

Over the next days, weeks, months, continue to practice these new ideas and movements by pulling up a mental picture ; bring him into it as he is when starting to be ugly. When you get the picture in mind, visualize gracefully pulling off these two tricks— Stretchy-Lip and Move Along!

Picture yourself doing a perfect Stretchy-Lip, then a smooth Move Along. Also see yourself feeling good about what you've accomplished!

> **Psych Note: This is the exact form of practice the**

> greatest athletes use. They visualize themselves doing the new thing, at first slowly, picking up speed with increasing familiarity and confidence. They also visualize seeing themselves being successful, then feeling good afterward.

* * *

MASTERY

Pull out one or two points from this chapter that you especially want to absorb fast and write them here. (Checking your MASTERY notes once a week strengthens their power to change you.)

1. _____

_____

2. _____

_____

Chapter 3

Relationship Problems: Are Yours Special?

"But don't all couples have these same problems?"

And this, "But we have more problems than just his drinking! What about those?"

I hear these questions at every workshop. Many of you probably are wondering the same.

The answer is "Yes, both of those are true." But the key word in the second response is "most," some of the same problems. All couples have problems. All people who interact at all will have problems; that's because each individual differs from others in few or many ways, so the problems that develop often are tied to those differences.

However, the major difference between your relationship problems and those of other, happier relationships, is in the number of problems you must deal with. A, of course, the way you deal with them. Another important difference is that few of their problems get as serious as yours do.

So yes, all couples have some of the same problems, but in a drinker's relationship there are more of them, and they tend to be more serious.

One factor contributing to this unhappy reality is that the problems that arise in your relationship tend to linger, and get worse. You may hesitate to address them because you want to avoid nuclear war, or he lays down the law as to the solution—which you know is guaranteed not to work. (You begin to remember that going by his rules is how you got here in the first place).

The most disturbing and painful problems are the emotional problems which, upon close examination, turn out to be little more than the effect of his bad behavior on you and the stress from the sheer number of problems that need to be resolved.

It's not because you're losing it either. What's happening to you results from specific bad behaviors in your partner. Much of his bad behavior turns out to create situations that are poison to your Manufacturer-installed wiring and not because you're different from other women. Females—human and animal—are factory-wired to react strongly to specific behaviors, behaviors known to go hand in hand with over-drinking. No, darlin', it's not you!

As to your problems, let's start by highlighting basic differences between healthy and not-so-healthy relationships. In many of your cases, you have responded in ways that would be considered normal reactions to the situation. That's not the issue right now; it's that most of you have not known much about the "rules" of healthy interactions.

And why is that? It's because most of you never learned the guidelines. Many of you never had the privilege of living with and daily observing two healthy adults working through their problems with love and respect.

Consequently, if you never observed it, how could you have known and become adept at using those healthy ways? Where would you have ever seen such things as patience with, and respect for, someone you disagree with?

Lacking these "rules," relationship problems tend to get resolved by one individual's wants rather than by the two of them, the relationship's needs. (Successful relationships, to be healthy, usually are only finalized after both parties are well acquainted with their own needs, and the needs, wants, and preferences of the other—as well as discovering whether the other party has the skills of problem-solving. Lacking these, the couple's chances for lasting happiness are slim.

Here's a starter on your journey to a full, happy, satisfying relationship—even if it's not with him.

Some Differences Between Healthy Relationships and Less Healthy Relationships

1. First, the number of problems on the table at the same time differs drastically. Many more problems arise in an over-drinker's relationships.

2. Next, the seriousness of your problems demands more mental, emotional, even physical energy from both of you than is the norm. Thus, while drinkers's relationships have the same problems as other relationships (plus problems other relationships do not have), those similar kinds of problems either

start out as more difficult where over-drinking is involved, or they become that way over time.

3. Having more problems (and more serious problems) inevitably results in these game breakers:

a. Problems that were serious to start with, and those that evolved to be more difficult, require far more energy and skill than over-drinkers have to work with. Combined with your lack of experience and expertise in these same skills, you have a dead end. Relationship problems are meant to be solved by a two-person team. In most drinkers's relationships, those things required to solve relationship and life problems simply are not part of the formula.

b. As the more serious problems build up more pressure, they tend to create still more problems, problems that wouldn't be there except for other problems that produced these new ones. (Stress effects from these problems throw both parties out of line, sometimes setting you up for serious illnesses, even mental health problems. All of these now become additional problems, extreme stressors. The pressure tends to be so great most of the time that both parties are robbed of their full intellectual ability to resolve them.

c. Both parties are steadily drained by the sheer number and weight of their problems, making it nearly impossible for both to focus on any one of them without being bombarded and torn away to deal with another that one gone into crisis mode.

4. The greatest difference between healthy and not-so-healthy relationships, however, is in the way problems are handled—or not. Take note of the following ways healthy relationships resolve problems.

* * *

Read over the following elements of a healthy relationship. Check any that you do not have in your relationship.

____ They don't call one another names.

____ They don't point the finger of blame. (Since both parties make mistakes and occasionally screw up, both keep in mind that any problems belong to both of them. They know that neither is perfect enough to blame the other. (Blame only pops up when one tries to put the blame-burden on the other.)

____ Partners in a healthy relationship listen carefully, respectfully to the other person's point of view, allowing each other to fully speak their ideas without interruption, and allow each other to speak their full piece.

____ These partners ask each other for opinions, then listen carefully, respectfully, staying open. They then respect a differing point of view.

____ A healthy partner will never put down the other person's point of view. If it gets hot, an issue can be rested, but only if an "appointment" is made to come back to it after each of you has time to think things through and settle down. (This technique prevents emotions from taking over, rather than the common sense that's needed.)

____ In a healthy relationship, partners ask one another about their "feelings" concerning the problem, as well as each proposed solution, both making sure they understand their partner's thinking. (They listen so well that they can repeat what has just been said, and often do just to be sure they got it right.)

____ Partners in healthy relationships rarely interrupt each other, waiting until their partner has finished speaking. (Some have been taught in couples's counseling to count to three before speaking. It's a good trick, it cuts down reflex anger responses.)

____ Patience with one another is primary. (Impatience is just the face of self-centeredness.)

____ In healthy relationships partners respectfully remind each other of any "rule" with gentleness (and humor where possible).

How many checkmarks do you have? _____

(Don't worry if you didn't check any: I didn't expect you to.) In fact, I put these concepts in to get your attention, for your enrichment, not to measure yourself by.

Simply thinking about these rules of healthy relationships is enough to gradually make them part of your own life—which is likely all that's going to change in this regard.

These "rules" aren't taught in school, for the most part; they are only learned by growing up in an environment where they are practiced. I have found that in most cases, neither the drinker or his woman were that lucky. Remembering this can help both maintain loving respect as they learn together—if the drinker is willing. And able. (Think: You would now be speaking Chinese if you had grown up in a home where Chinese was spoken. That's how most life skills are learned—a childhood filled with good examples.) Fortunately, like a second language, these rules can be learned at any time in life. It takes only willingness. And a bit more work than it would have been if you had received it on the first go-around.

Oh, My, Yes! You Surely Have More Problems Than Just the Drinking

Yes, you surely have other problems: Money problems, job problems, health problems, relationship problems, anger problems, jealousy problems, social problems, sexual problems, sexual misbehavior, and oh lord that hair!

All love relationships run into some of these, but usually not at crisis levels, and not stacked up, coming only one at a time.

In the over-drinker's relationships, for all the reasons we've been discussing, problems sit there, accumulating into a mass of unresolved problems, growing heavier and more alarming by the day. You are likely hampered by now with wounded emotions that will interfere with your mental clarity, making it difficult to discuss problems. If he blows up when you talk about a problem, if he refuses to learn these rules, you may as well drop it. You'll get no progress. Still, if you choose to stay with this man (or find another), you must learn these ways of resolving problems or you will see the same conditions arising again and again.

If your relationship is complicated by over-drinking, problems will continue to block you. New problems, old problems. There is no escaping this because at least one half of your team is severely limited. As he deteriorates, you will see your problems increase. They won't just go away if you ignore them.

At some point, both parties become overwhelmed: He—by what his drinking is doing to his brain and life; by what your experiences with him are doing to your brain and life. His judgement begins to fail; indeed, his brain is diminished iin all areas where intelligent thought occurs. It's as if you are plowing a rough field while dragging a crippled ox.

Furthermore, your judgement and clarity (and everything else, by the way) is affected, diminished by emotional pain, anger, frustration, and most especially by self-condemnation and its consequent lowered self-esteem.

The Good News: Each of those things is totally fixable, so accept that there's a bucketful of hope here.

While most of your relationship problems occur because of what his drinking is causing and the lack of skills no one ever taught either of you, that doesn't mean you should have so much compassion for him that you lay your own life on the altar. In healthy relationships that face problems, often one sacrifices for another, but then the other sacrifices at approximately the same rate. (No one keeps score, but you have to keep a rudimentary idea of the score, else you will be abusively taken advantage of.) In dealing with an over-drinker, your sacrifices are for what is most likely a lost cause.

Even so, the typical drinker's woman will feel obligated to sacrifice herself, perhaps for what she believes is love, perhaps because she's been taught that a woman must do this.

While she may be angry at him, she takes on the failure to resolve problems as her personal failure. Let's halt that right now! Who is your best friend?

Right—it's yourself. If she doesn't take care of you, you aren't going to do very well at anything.

Most women I've worked with have said something like this: "It's not just the drinking. We've got a lot of other problems besides his drinking—and some are even worse! We don't ever have any fun together, we hardly ever have sex, our financial condition is desperate. And I think he may be cheating on me."

I don't doubt that these other problems seem worse than just the drinking. If you don't accept that his drinking (which includes the effect it has on him) underlies almost all of the problems you just told me about.

Life hands all of us loads of problems: the economy goes bad; people we love get sick or die; it rains too much, it rains too little; work is too demanding or you can't find any, and what to do with this hair? But here are the facts of life: A drinking problem is in a problem class of its own.

What gives it that special status? Because it's a problem that actually creates more problems and worsens others. Some of those problems can seem worse than the drinking, but the drinking is just sitting there producing this and steadily producing other problems. Some of those problems stress you to the point of illness, others can rip your heart out; some lay waste to parts of your life, but what they all have in common is this: They would not exist(at least this bad) if he didn't over-drink.

If not a direct result of a drinking bout, then indirectly, such as trouble on a job from slipping performance or poor attendance, or loss of that job, resulting now in financial pressures that crush you. Each of those problems carry serious separate problems in them—for instance, the lack of a healthy diet because of loss of income.

Your Problem Pile from Another Perspective

Let's go back to that basement full of problems. In the next three or four minutes, list as many of them as you can think of. Ten would be nice, but three may be enough to give you the benefit of this eye-opening exercise. While most of the time you try to get these problems off your mind, now is the time to spotlight them so take a minute or three to ponder them, then you can pack them away again.

List the first problem that comes to mind, then the next, and then the next. The listing process may jump-start your brain's problem center, so don't be surprised it they start flowing once you begin. Go ahead and list as many as you can think of.

What's the first relationship problem that comes to mind?

1. _____

And the next?

2. _____

And the next:

3. _____
And so on:

4. _____

5. _____

6. _____

7. _____

8. _____

9. _____

10. _____

    Even if you only listed a few problems right now, you've done well enough for our purposes here; normally, to go about your day, you have learned to shut the door on the problems you're now pulling up to look at. But it's another important element of changing everything in your life, so please be patient and make your list. Add others either in the Note Pages in the back of this book, or in your journal or notebook.

    Once you've made your list, this is a good time to take a break.
    Get a sip of tea, take a bathroom break, walk around the block. Come back as soon as you feel the relief: What we get into next can totally change your life. It will certainly change the way you understand your life.

* * *

Great, you're back!
Ready to get back to work?
Very Good! Let's get to it.

In that last exercise, how many problems did you list? _____. (We'll use this number to change the way you see your whole life with this man.)

1. Read over the first problem you listed; now ask whether any part of that problem is due to, or even associated with, his drinking. If so, circle its number. Continue down your list and do the same for each problem listed.
2. How many problems did you circle? _____

Now, complete the following statements using the numbers you've come up with.

"Of the _____ problems I listed, _____ of them are tied to his drinking."

Excellent. Now read that sentence again—out loud.

Next, take the same numbers, and say the same thing but in another way.

"If he quit drinking, _____ of the _____ problems I listed would improve—or disappear."

Now read that sentence out loud.

What emotions do these words stir up?

___Sadness?
___Anger?
___Depressed?
___Hopeless?
___Happy (because now you're seeing the light!)

___Other_____
_____

Has this exercise brought you a stronger sense of what's going on in your life?

Yes   No

After doing these exercises and going about the other things in your life, you may think of other problems you didn't list. When that happens, come back and add them to this list, then re-calculate your numbers and read aloud your new statements.

Fact
Whatever causes a problem IS a problem.

Fact
If your relationship problems are connected to his drinking, then his drinking is problem drinking.

Most women, upon seeing that many (most?) of their relationship (and life) problems trace back to their mate's drinking feel a mental shift. If you feel this, stay with it; savor it. You are engraving truth; it becomes an understanding that won't slip away under pressure—and it will change your life.

Seeming to be saying something negative, this insight will change your life in a very positive way. As you understand any problem better, solutions easier slip into place. Learning something Bad turns out to be Good.

With a better understanding of your situation, solutions you come up with now various problems will be more accurately enacted. That means they will be more effective.

Another Very Important Point
If a number of your relationship problems are associated with *his* drinking, then no matter what he says, *you* can't be the problem!

* * *

Your outcome on this exercise also shows you that no matter who his partner might be, her problems right now would be exactly the same as those you just listed.

(If he runs to another woman, citing your failures as the

"reason" for the failed relationship, be assured that she will soon be slammed with all the same problems you have had, and she'll be stressing exactly like you. Maybe worse, because over-drinkers inexorably keep getting worse. You get your revenge.

Grin.

> **Psych Note:** Sanity is defined and judged by whether a person's behavior hurts him or someone else. When one's behavior causes harm to someone he says cares for, yet he doesn't stop that behavior, it's not sane.
>
> Or else he really doesn't care about her. That's a hard idea for some of you to look at, but if it's true, the sooner you accept it, the sooner your pain will end.

A certain level of doing harm to oneself or others causes the doer to be confined, locked away—in a mental institution or jail. Once confined, almost all will soon vow they've changed, that they've learned their lesson.

Most of them will truly believe they have changed as the result of this experience (which is why they can be so convincing). Likely, he will be upset if you don't jump on his bandwagon. This, in itself, proof that he really hasn't changed: He's still demanding that the world (you) conform itself to whatever he says or thinks.

The cure for your emotional reactions to this scene: Step back and check out who is locked up. (It's not you.) If his problems are even close to this bad, hen you, my sweet, simply cannot be the problem—as he has worked so hard to make you believe.

Unless you see *lots* of evidence of any claimed change, the change you are looking for won't last. Don't be fooled by "jailhouse repentance." Do not rely on any claimed change being permanent until at least a year has passed without his slipping back to some of the old ways. (Even after a year, you can never be sure . . . .)

This suggests that you resist believing his assertion that he has changed, no matter how sincere he seems, or how upset he gets when you don't excitedly jump on board. Remember that his getting upset because you don't fall for it is simply *proof* that he has not changed.

If you were buying a used car, you'd try it out thoroughly. Your safety, your life depend on the fitness of the car. Much more must you hold back latching onto his claims that he's learned his lesson. You can let him back in (if he's not violent), but not back into your emotions. At least not until he's proved himself.

Oh, in the case of violence, only one in about a thousand will stay quit. Your safety, your life, your beauty, depend on knowing this and heeding it.

Sadly, true change, lasting change, is only the case less than 10 percent of the time in the case of drinking. Would you ride in a car that was only 10 percent sure of being stable?

When a person is fooling himself, he is, at the very least, temporarily insane. His mind is basing its stand on a fantasy, something that is not real. That is very like the thinking of the schizophrenic disorder. The drinker maintains belief in something that's not real—his true condition.

This means you can sanely and confidently back off from taking anything he says seriously until you have a mass of proof, actions! Not just his words.

"What you *do* is so loud I can't hear what you say!"

You don't need to make a show of it; just follow that guideline. His brain is no longer working normally; consequently, you cannot base your life, your future, welfare, your day on whatever he says or claims at the moment.

Imagine now how much time and emotional grief you will save yourself with this new guideline. Ah! You may get the energy to begin building yourself a more satisfying, rewarding life.

Or start getting one.

* * *

What if Nothing Happens When He Drinks?

Every once in awhile, I hear this: "But nothing bad happens when he drinks. He's what you might call a happy drunk."

My answer to that is, "If *nothing* happens when he drinks, do the two of you grow closer, as healthy couples do?"

If a relationship isn't growing, it's dying.

If you fight and argue when he drinks, you're obviously moving farther apart. If you get frustrated, angry, or hurt by the things he says or does, you're obviously moving farther apart. Less obvious perhaps is that when he leaves you alone to go have fun or just drink, or isolates himself, you're moving further apart.

In other words, when it seems like nothing happens in your relationship, something *is* happening. Stagnation, starvation, death.

Relationships (like plants) shrivel if they are not tended regularly. No relationship can survive ongoing shrinkage—not a business relationship, a family relationship, a friendship, and definitely not a love relationship. Relationships aren't like works of art that come into being, then just remain the same. Relationships are like plants, like your spirit: they require regular water and feeding; otherwise, gradual shriveling and death.

Research shows that happy lifelong relationships are built on doing things together, both good things and hard things, working and playing and crying together. Surprising to many is the finding that when couples work together to resolve a problem is when the strongest bonds are formed. The relationship deepens.

Every time a couple join forces they strengthen their bond. It's the working together, especially through the hard times, leaning on one another, holding each other up, each using his or her unique skills to assist the other, bring a solution. Appreciating each other's deepens the relationship.

Pushing away problems, hiding from the uncomfortable, perhaps from fear they will damage the relationship—those things will eventually destroy it.

A Drinker's Limited Opportunities for Change

It's not as if he has every day of the rest of his life to change. Some of the most important (yet largely ignored) research on over-drinking shows that the majority of the very few lasting fixes occur during only two very short periods in the progression of a drinking problem. It's not as most suppose, that the drinker will "see the light" at any point in his downslide.

Even in those two, fairly short, openings, his chances of making it out of his mess are still extremely slim. Let's dig a little further:

In the unavoidable progression of over-drinking, the only times we see the drinker recognizing his problem and effectively responding are

--The Early Stage, and
--The Late-Middle Stage.

Early On: Some men are reached at the very start of drinking too much. (Remember that what makes it "too much" is that problems arise from it.) A few men are, in the Early Stage, receptive to information, education about drinking. In all my research, the results on drinking from this education are all I've ever found that actually stopped (or delayed) the onset of more serious drinking.

The successful outcomes of forced education, such as driving school as part of the penalty for driving under the influence, stands as proof to all that if there is a "line" where one crosses into a drinking problem, it's way back there in the earliest Early Stage.

National statistics reveal that a large number of men forced into driving school because of drunk driving charges do not repeat the drunk driving. At least not for two years these studies follow up.

No, that's not very promising, yet it does establish a certain openness that is not there shortly after as he progresses.

These findings, by far the most optimistic I've run across, must be used to identify drinkers just starting to go over "the line," to educate you and them (and professionals) to the effect on their bodies and brains. The cost will produce greater gains.

But education alone is of little or no use beyond the Early Stage. Only before and during early phases is the drinker able to act on it.

Two years without driving drunk—or being caught driving drunk—isn't recovery. On the other hand, it is evidence that, at the onset of trouble associated with drinking, many can and do achieve control (either control of their drinking or control of not driving). And this is not the case afterward. No form of treatment invented so far produces the same results.

Whether the driver is not re-arrested on a drinking charge or not rearrested because he never drives after one drink, and he mostly stays home—whichever it is demonstrates that he still has a significant amount of personal—in this Early Stage. Before the brain damage has eaten away his Judgement Center and Behavior Control Center.

These findings are backed up by showing that drinking drivers who don't attend these classes do have a significant number of repeat arrests on drinking or drug charges in the following two years.

A drinking problem gone too far is about losing personal power to change. A staggering amount of personal power is required to make a turn-around. It requires being able to see problems and gain skills to respond to them without drinking, and all the grounded physical and mental ability to maintain those changes. It takes an incredible amount of brain power.

And that is precisely what is being lost with every drink.

Early on, an over-drinker's brain is still functioning well enough to do that. When given knowledge of their disorder and the unavoidable end of the path they're on, many early stage over-drinkers muster their personal forces and change direction. But this period of openness and sufficient ability appears to be limited. It clearly appears that when those brain changes make even a small dent, the drinker's ability to follow through on desired changes diminishes. At least until-

Very Late in His Disintegration: The only other time there seems to be much hope of change is some five to twenty years later—for him and for you. The five to twenty depends on how much he drinks and how fast he deteriorates.

Again, the great tragedy of our current approach to drinking disorders is that it takes five to 20 years for an over-drinker to develop some of the visible signs that professionals are required to find in order to diagnose big trouble with drinking.

Currently, an over-drinker must have that diagnosis of a drinking problem to get treatment. (No insurance pays for treatment unless the required signs are present. We can all begin to address this with the powers that be at every opportunity.)

A further crimp in diagnosis of drinking problems is that it depends almost totally upon—believe it or not—what we call "self report." That means the diagnosis is based on what the drinker tells the professional! In all the world, an over-drinker is the least trustworthy assessor and reporter of his own drinking behavior.

What Should We Professionals Do With the Knowledge We Already Possess?

We professionals can begin to address these issues, especially the problem of not being allowed to diagnose a drinking problem until it's in its last stages. Catching it in the last stages prevents fixing it for the mass of cases. We practitioners can insist on expanding the number and type of signs to watch for—as well as start to push for getting access to treatment earlier in the disorder. Much earlier.

Indeed, insurance companies might jump on board as we look at the money that could be saved: A part-time treatment early on is often sufficient, a solution that doesn't keep the patient from work, and doesn't cost the insurance company so much. (As with any other disorder, this approach is certain to be more effective than any other form of treatment coming later.) Research shows that none of them work very well. (Since it involves mostly education and just a tad of psychology, early treatment will cost far, far less than what is required later. Listen up, insurance companies!)

Each of you readers can share the information here with others, whether or not they personally live with the problem; build a larger group saying that we must not wait for a drinker to become a staggering drunk, or until he kills an entire family in an auto accident to say Wow! Now he qualifies for intensive treatment.

The easiest glitch to fix in our current cultural stance toward alcohol is to institute education about alcohol, its effects of thinking and behavior and why—the effects it has on the body (especially the brain). This education must be applied before Middle School—where so many youngsters start moving off-track.

The serious effects on brain cells is especially staggering in young people. If young people learn, pre-teens, the realities of drinking alcohol and its physical effects, they are better equipped to make better choices.

If we don't teach them—**long before they <u>need</u> to know it**—they will continue to be lured to the path that seems most exciting. Educating the young—at school, surrounded by peers—will erase much of the lure. There is much money and power behind production and sales of alcohol, and much cultural ignorance of the facts, so it may not be easy—but it must begin.

Now "The Late Stage," the next phase of over-drinking where a drinker has a chance of being open to treatment. But it won't come for five to twenty years after the problem becomes evident. If he hasn't been able to stop up until now, that's not going to change. And, as you're seeing, with every drink, his ability to stop diminishes.

By the Late Stage, he has admitted, even to himself, that he has a problem; he simply cannot stop (or more accurately, he cannot stay stopped). He has by now established and accepted that he cannot do without the feeling that only alcohol gives him.

By Late Stage, he has stopped stopping after hundreds of failed attempts. And yes we count all those hung-over mornings when he swore he was done. Additionally, many can no longer sustain their drinking (either financially or health-wise).

(I believe that the biggest reason he is more likely to seek early help is that it's the only time he will be allowed to get it by the powers that decide such things. A plus is that it likely will avoid the stigma, being popularly considered a lesser problem.)

Diagnosis of an alcohol problem, admission to treatment, and insurance payments for that treatment, all require signs that accompany a deteriorated body and brain. Late Stage signs. Signs that the brain is already greatly deteriorated. (Sufficiently deteriorated, we can see, to diminish his chances of of ever making it, even with the best of help—of which there is precious little available to any but the very rich.)

Instituting earlier diagnosis will change all of that.

So how does all of this information impact you, the drinker's woman?

You are the person who is the most impacted and harmed by those very long five to twenty years of continued drinking and misbehavior before a drinker arrives at his last likely opportunity to break free. But by then, you may not care anymore.

Those very long five to twenty years of living with bad and worse behavior devastate a drinker's partner, except, that is, if she has a new bag of tricks and a strong support system.

And that's what you need: A new bag of tricks and a strong support system. If those previously close to you don't support you in any changes you decide to make, then put a little distance between them and you until you are settled and strong again. Take care of yourself; no one else will.

It turns out that the very misbehaviors alcohol can create (through specific brain changes) produce the worst sort of damage to a woman—because of her emotional wiring. Her home (nest) is shaken loose; her brood's welfare is threatened. His absence (physical and emotional) puts incredible pressure on her. The loss of his partnership turns her world over, and all the weight of it slides onto her.

The stress and emotional abuse she endures take a horrible toll. And worse: Her options are depleted.

She's older—five to twenty years older.

She's likely mentally and physically harmed.

(The word "Amen!" is said to mean "Pay attention to that!" I would like you to take every *   *   * as my saying "Amen!")

Should you think that enduring five to twenty more years of

what's going on now isn't so bad, remember that as long as he continues to drink any alcohol, he will continue to get worse.

But he won't even stay as bad as he is. He will get worse. More ugliness; more bad behavior.

What's likely to happen to you if what I say is true?

Very little good. Unless, that is, you get the help you need to change the way you react to him and his stuff, and reestablish a satisfying life. Even then, you cannot escape the fallout of his progressive disorder if you live with him. His worsening health and his worsening behavior will disrupt and damage everything.

The impact on a drinker's woman through all of the stages of over-drinking is far greater than most suppose. And the worst of it appears to occur during those five to twenty in-between years, he's clearly got a problem, but no one (especially him) is willing to do anything about it. This is when he's behaving his worst; it will be in just those areas that most damage a woman.

After those five to twenty bad years, the drinker's woman—one of nature's strongest creatures—burns out, wears out, gives up. That burn-out occurs long before the drinker qualifies for treatment. Unfortunately, reading this book now suggests that the man in question is probably already behaving badly enough that to be at least in the Middle Stages (likely Late Middle).

The Good News: You are not alone. Very few people, drinkers or their women, register what is happening until way past Early Stage. By the time his woman begins looking for help, the drinker has already made a number of attempts to control both his drinking and his behavior. And those attempts, no matter how determined he is, will have failed—or you wouldn't be here.

Likely you are in for years and years more of increasingly bad behavior. These harsh facts are not publicized, and the consequent lack of common awareness has resulted in millions of women (as many as 20 to 30 million at the time of this writing) continue living in hell—right here, in the United States alone. Their hell is either coping with an over-drinker who is present or coping with their own mental and emotional condition resulting from the very real abuses over-drinkers dump on their women.

Based on news reports from around the world, the number of affected women in the United States appears to be matched by those in most countries of the world. From the Far East: China, Thailand, Korea, to Africa :Kenya, Libya, South Africa—all report problems with increasing over-drinking. The result is untold suffering of untold millions of women. As you read this, near a million women right there in in your state, your area, survive in their private and lonely hell. Most keep on keeping on because they either hold the fantasy that one day he's going to change—or they have numbed themselves so thoroughly that they just don't feel anything anymore.

Perhaps worse, most of these women believe are at least partly responsible for the drinking and also the bad behavior. Believing she is somewhat to blame, coupled with his increasingly disrespectful treatment of her, she loses self-esteem, self-confidence, and most of her enjoyment of life.

Of course, you are learning that she has failed because she aimed too many of her shots at the wrong targets—the problems that were produced by the source problem. Time spent on getting him home on time, on investigating whether he's cheating. These targets have fooled her into wasting all her ammunition with little or no positive effect.

And of course, a handful of people have become very, very rich by leaving everything as it is, while millions upon millions are wretched.

Whew! It's About Time for More Good News

- The tricks you pick up here are going to help you control, rebuild, reshape your own life. You'll have the energy to do that once you've stopped trying to fix him. You may be able to stay in place if that's your choice, and "live around" his problem, but stay or go, you are laying the foundation of a dramatic and positive personal life change.

- Once you absorb the information in this book, you can be free—go back to being your best self.
- Once you learn what his manipulation tricks are, and use these new ways to avoid or counteract them, he won't be able to manipulate, overwhelm, or bully you the way he has.

- Once you understand what's really going on with him, you no longer carry a sense of guilt or shame for being a failure. You clearly realize it's not you—it's him who is messed up.

- All these things hugely increases your joy in life—and freedom to be who you really are, a dynamite gal.

More on What's Happening to Him

Due to malfunctioning body parts, alcohol affects this man differently than it does most other people. His body doesn't adequately process (break down) the alcohol in his blood. That means it stays in his system longer than it does in others—and it stays at a higher strength than in others. This is why brain and other bodily damage speed up over time.

Rapidly entering his bloodstream, alcohol rushes to his brain, arriving in seconds. Every second it remains in him, moving in the blood from organ to organ, it affects, sedates, damages, and kills the cells of his body—notably his brain cells.

As soon as a brain cell is touched (within seconds of the alcohol getting in his mouth it enters his bloodstream, rapidly swirling through his body and affecting every single body cell it touches—and its effect begins. (That's why you can almost always tell if he's had even one drink. You've seen it so many times, the way alcohol affects him is as familiar as your feet. Believe me, if you suspect he's been drinking, he has.)

He may be puzzled and amazed that you can tell so quickly. He usually will adamantly tell you that you're crazy. But you're not. He may have said such things often enough to instill self-doubt in you. Especially will you have begun to doubt your perceptions. But be assured: Your body-brain is clear and unaffected by a drug; he's the one off-kilter.

The changes in his brain and body tissues cause specific physical changes, specific changes in his body movements, and in his speech; mental changes that affect his personality begin with his first swallow. That first damage slam will be repeated and repeated and repeated for as long as any molecules of alcohol are left in his blood.

Since the kind of change these effects create become more pronounced with each cell contact with the alcohol consider: Of course you can see them; of course you can recognize them from their very first effects. The same changes you see after just one drink just become more pronounced until everyone else would agree that he's drunk. The same body-brain parts are affected more with each drink.

As his drinking problem progresses, these effects become more severe: thought process, physical functions, slurring, loss of emotional control. Around then comes loss of bladder control—and worse. You may dread the way they appear finally, but the effects began the first seconds after he took the first sip. Slip back into your self-confidence: You are not imagining things. If you suspect he's had a drink, then you've been picking up on small clues, and almost certainly he has.

Brain areas first hit by the stun-damage-then-kill effect are most pertinently the areas of brain where his judgement, planning, decision-making, and self-control center. Slammed soonest by the ongoing flow of alcohol in his blood, his brain continues to be bombarded with altering effects until every molecule of alcohol has been broken down and ejected from his body. If he's had only two 8-ounce beers, or two 5-ounce glasses of wine, or two small shots, it takes at least an hour and a half for the destructive effect to let up.

What can you do about any of that? _____

Can you fix any part of it and make it stay fixed? _____

Can you begin now to stop trying to fix it (him)? _____

Always Keep in Mind the Source Problem
Keeping the source problem—his drinking—firmly in mind from now on will make your ride much smoother. It's getting wrapped up in the events, his accusations, and your own self-condemnation that put the most stress on you. Firmly remembering just what's going on will make all the difference.

Over-drinking likes to pretend it's the natural result of a bad childhood, or a bad day, or any number of unfortunate experiences—or a flat tire, a hangnail, or a snoot full of snuff. He uses these excuses—why? Because they work! Now you're about to change how well these old tricks work using your new tricks.

He sees all his many problems as justifying his drinking, not as causing or worsening them. But you will no longer be fooled. The problems he claims make him drink are pretty much the same as for all the rest of human-kind, but all of them aren't over-drinking.

To sum up: His problem is his drinking, the problems it creates, and what it is doing to his mind. Your problem is how all of that affects you.

Until the underlying problem, his drinking, is resolved, few of your other relationship problems will be.

Psych Note: Some of your really wonderful qualities are

what create and maintain the trap that has been sprung on you. But that doesn't mean those qualities are bad; don't condemn those qualities! They are excellent qualities.

You got trapped, not by your qualities but by a flawed partner; you've been trapped into spending yourself trying to fix him. You have worked to ease his discomfort, ease his emotional pain, calm his turmoil, cheer him up, and clean up after him. Rather than appreciate it, he came to demand it—and resent it Now, if you don't serve up on demand those parts of yourself that actually were gifts to him, he punishes you by flying into rages, name-calling, and the like.

Solution: Don't throw good energy on top of mistreated energy. The easiest way to redirect your efforts is to focus all your super qualities and know-how on rebuilding your own life! On learning tricks to avoid falling back into emotional slavery.

Every time you catch yourself pondering how to change something in him or fix a problem his drinking has created, pull out your list of wonderful things you are going to do with your own life and turn your intelligence and talent in that direction. This will pay off. Big! Spending yourself on trying to please someone who never will be pleased—at least not for long—is just no longer part of your life plan.

The extra energy you spend on him does no good anyway. Has it? It doesn't please him—not for long anyway, and it surely doesn't please you. As you retreat from doing cleanup and tip-toeing around his sensitivities, you will find a truckload of mental and emotional energy. How will you spend it? Decide that now and it will flow easier when you get there.

One way to do this is to take the "quiet time" or "something fun" time and focus it onto planning the next step toward one of your dreams.

Call that college and ask for a class schedule. Make an appointment with a college counselor to research adding more skills and knowledge to your already stellar package. Or you can throw yourself into your job or hobbies—and when they don't give you pleasure and reward, start looking for a new job or new hobbies.

You will use the "something fun" times for paging through news magazines to find women you would like to be more like. Begin listing the qualities you see in them that you want for yourself, find people in your regular life with qualities you would like to have (or get back). Be around those people as much as possible and imitate the good quality you admire. You must build in time for recovering from a tense situation; let's fill the time with things that will greatly benefit you or bring you joy.

A Man of Many Sorrows

You (and others) may feel sorry for him because of his bad childhood, his war wounds, or his bad day, resulting in letting him get away with bad behavior.

If anyone presses him about his bad behavior, he reminds them of his special difficulties. He learned long ago to inform others of his sufferings let him slide right off of the hot seat.

You are wonderfully compassionate, and he has used (consciously or not) that compassion to get by with unacceptable behavior. This doesn't suggest your compassion is a fault, or that you are stupid. On the other hand, women *without* your high level of compassion long ago packed their bags and moved along.

None of this is to say that whatever he has suffered is petty; but many people carry the same wounds, yet they do not drink away all the goodness in their lives, or drink to the extent they wound those they claim to love.

As to his many problems, his real problem isn't any of the things it hides behind. His problem is not having bad days, bad luck, bad childhood. (A recovering priest who calls himself Father John Doe wrote that all the things an over-drinker claims "make" him drink are not "causes" at all—merely occasions. Occasions for him to drink and over-drink, and to feel justified doing it. Better yet, the "causes" of his drinking serve to keep most others off his back.)

No one can complain louder or longer about the things that have happened to him. While he presents them as being bad, he actually treasures and hoards up incidents of bad luck or bad treatment. He stores them for future use, ammunition to blast anyone who dares try to make him accountable for his behavior.

Sadly, most people buy it. Including you. Until now.

> **Psych Note:** While almost all over-drinkers relapse and quickly get back to the way things were, I've never known of a drinker's woman, once she got a firm hold on this new way of living, who ever went back to her old ways.

So—how about you go do something fun. Just because you

can!

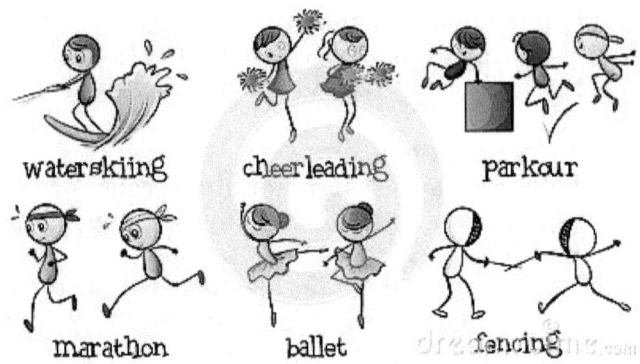

When you feel tense, take a deep, deep breath and let your shoulders drop. Most people can spot their tension rising by the tightening in their shoulders and neck. Take a deep breath, and relax (best you can at the moment, your new rule for most any situation: Just do the best you can under the circumstances of the moment). Let your shoulders relax, then your neck. Now it's safer to think about things you want to accomplish or do or maybe learn, ever in your life. Think of dreams you've had for your life or livelihood whose ideas still stir you.

Begin a "living list," one you keep open forever to add new ideas or for scratching one out. Look for your dreams to list all the way back to childhood. I always wanted to take ballet classes—but was unable. Our family was old-fashioned, strict Baptist where dancing was considered a sin. Did you want to learn ballet? To play the piano? Speak French? Be a makeup artist? A seamstress? Go back to school and get a certification or degree? Become an archeologist? A nurse? A doctor? To hang-glide, or bungie-jump, or pilot an airplane? Did you want to be a counselor? If any of those fire a spark, even a tiny one, go ahead and list that thing.

Be sure to add to this list all the things you enjoy doing now. Bike-riding, sewing, dancing, making a garden, reading, creating something lovely, making jewelry, talking with a friend, sex, walking the beach, finishing up the ironing, writing a book, becoming a perfectly organized person, blowing glass, repainting your living room . . . .

Below is a place to start, right now while the sparks are still warm.

Don't nix any idea; it if pops to mind, go ahead and write it. You won't be charged extra for things that you later decide to scratch!

Activities You Would Like to Do
(Be sure to include activities you enjoy doing now, not just those you want for the future.)

1. _____

2. _____

3. _____

4. _____

5. _____

Copy this list into a special notebook or journal (or the Note Pages at the back of this book). Simply starting a list will spark your subconscious; it loves this kind of exercise because thoughts of these things create a sweet chemistry in the brain.

Prioritize items by their appeal to you right now. Next, pull out three to five of what seem to be the best and set up in your notebook a page for each item. On that page, begin a list of the steps you can think of right now that you'll need to take to gain that goal.

Too often in your life, I'll wager, you've let a dream fall by the wayside because someone said something negative about it—or because your circumstances blocked it. For the Beautiful Child inside you who is ready to fly, start writing a list of fun things to do.

When walking by a store, a thought may pop up: "You know, I'd love to get involved in (whatever it is you see that triggers the thought)." Dance lessons to Tai Chi. Whatever. List 'em!

This exercise is a giant step toward unfolding, restoring your true, beautiful self. And getting to know her better, who you really are—without doubt a lovely, creative being.

Now list at least three things you really want to achieve in your lifetime. Let's define "achieve" as "earning something." This list would include any classes or education or training you'd like to get; you may have already listed some of them but write them here anyway. It places a special emphasis.

What's important here is creating a focus list to come back to again and again when you can't immediately think of something fun and engrossing to do. Here's a spot for you to crack the shell and pop out more ideas.

A Starter List of Things You'd Like to Achieve

1. _____

2. _____

3. _____

Copy this Starter List into your journal too. (Another form of repetition, the key to making these ideas stick.) Doing this leaves you space to continue adding items every time you think of a new one. Later, perhaps once a year, you can go back over your list and scratch items or put them on the shelf. Each item on your "living lists" should have the power to grab your focus, to be so intriguing as to light up a vision of you doing or being that.

Turns out that even listing these items can produce thoughts that produce feelings lifting your spirits pretty high.

If a dream or goal or item to achieve turn up on both lists, well, that tells you something about how strong that dream is, tells you something about yourself too, about who you really are.

Next—you memorize the top three things on each of the two lists. This becomes another potent tool in your new Bag of Tricks.

Memorizing them, so you can test yourself several times a day and recite them, guarantees you will have easy access to the items even under stress.

You will have access even when you are anxious or depressed; these lists and the feelings they have the power to produce are natural healing medicines.

Stressed? Upset? Obsessing? Bored? Just pull off one item from one of these two lists and pay attention to what happens to you emotionally. Note any mood shift.

These lists only carry power when plugged in, like an

appliance. They don't work until you plug them in—think about them.

You Have Total Control Of What Stays in Your Mind

You can only focus on one thing at a time. No two thoughts can claim your attention at the same time.

When you wish to dump a thought, simply find another one to center on. It's that simple.

What's hard is doing it when you need to.

Memorization of two or three items from a list make it sure you will easily jump from the troubling thought to one of those.

Thoughts that bring you down are simply replaced. Thoughts of self-condemnation are easily dumped once you recall at least one special good thing about yourself.

Ejecting thoughts is much too hard. Replacing them is easy.

This trick works well in a multitude of situations: when an argument is brewing, when he says something mean and you feel compelled to respond Stop! Pull up an item from one of your lists (any of your lists is enough to do the **Thought-Dump Trick.**

Seeming difficult at first, right quickly your subconscious recognizes it for the solid pleasure it produces. At that point, you can quit working to do this; your subconscious does the work now, keeps your lists at the ready.

Once you stop expecting yourself to be perfect (demanding it), you make great headway.

Don't forget to continue rewarding yourself just for *trying* new things, not waiting for perfect performances. A simple loving pat on your own back (or butt) while telling yourself what a Good Girl you are is powerful.

Pat yourself on the butt! "You really *are* a good girl!"

The Tiny Surprise Trick
(This may become your most effective trick!)

Occasionally, in times of stress while in his company, do something odd, especially in response to his negativity; make it something unexpected. You want to learn how to create surprise at different levels. Here are some starter tricks to try out and evaluate their power. Then classify them accordingly in your coping catalogue.

A few examples to start your own "living" repertoire.

- Fish in your pocket for a quarter, or nickel, then hand it to him as if in passing, and Move Along;
- Bend over, find a dust bunny, stick it in your hair and Move Along;
- Give out the old evil laugh, WHAA-HA-HA! Then Move Along.
- Flip your skirt up high and kick out a can-can dance. (Let your Inner Actress enjoy this.)

The magic of a Tiny Surprise Trick arises because of what you do is unexpected, *and unusual.*

Unexpected events tend to freeze others in their mental tracks—briefly. We'll call this the Short Brain Freeze. The Short Brain Freeze lasts long enough to start a brisk Move Along.

Now go do something more fun than the argument he's fishing for. How about . . .

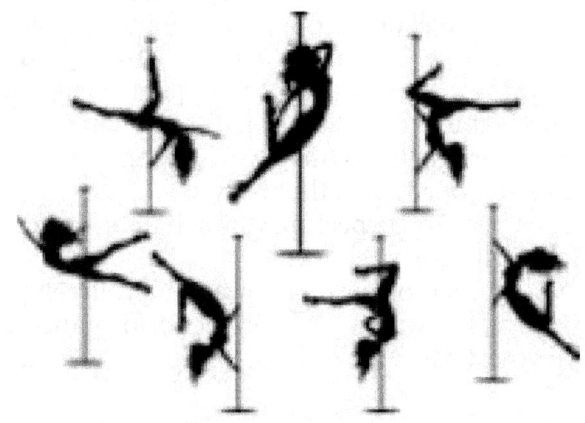

MASTERY

Pull out one or two points from this chapter that you especially want to absorb fast and write them here. (Checking your MASTERY notes once a week strengthens their power to change you.)

1. _____

_____

2. _____

_____

Chapter 4

Where you find out
> *Why you shut out clues you saw early on*
> *Why it's so hard to let go*
> *How to see better next time*

Did You See the Switch?
From Handsome Prince To Horse's Butt?

(Note: My calling your lover a Horse's Butt is not out of disrespect; it simply describes the form his disorder takes. Just as measles shows itself by breaking out in itchy spots, over-drinking shows itself by breaking out in Horse's Butt.)

Was He Always Like This?

Of course he wasn't! How do I know that? I know how smart you are, that you didn't fall in love with a Horse's Butt.

You fell in love with a great guy—cute, funny, sweet.

But then, he changed. Gradually. Gradually becoming what he is today.

I Saw it! . . . So Why Didn't I See it?"

"Why didn't I see it?" and "I should have known!" How many times have I heard these words? Hundreds of times? Thousands of times?

"I saw him do this stuff a long time ago," I hear now in my counseling office, "but I just ignored it or made excuses for it."

This is what drinkers's women say to themselves—for years, then finally to their therapist. They have intentionally beaten themselves up emotionally with such memories.

But how 'bout you add these two thoughts to your thought stash:

1. You originally fell in love with a man who, at the time, was sensitive, funny, fun, and romantic—at least most of the time;

2. Over-drinkers don't become Horse's Butts overnight; they gradually slip into it. (I guess we can make a funny here and say he gradually slipped into a Horse's Butt.)

When things happen gradually, they are hard to "see." Your eyes pick them up, but your brain's filtering system classifies them as insignificant. Think weight gain, wrinkles. bad hair. You don't see that new gram of superfat that just landed on your thighs, that wrinkle sinking a micrometer deeper. We're wired not to pay attention to minimal changes, otherwise we'd be overwhelmed with every shift in nature.

This means that we generally don't see gradual change (in anything) until it becomes something we can't miss. (Until we see ourselves in a store window and wonder who the chubby woman is, or instantly assume the glass must be warped, the experience of yours truly.)

Not only do people (and animals) usually not register small changes, but a form of denial further filters, and can block awareness of an unwanted change. This surely was wired in for the same reasons we're wired not to attend to every teensy change. Most of the time, this wiring is an aid to survival. But not when it's a cat creeping toward your nest, or when it's your dream of love getting slightly uglier.

You saw all of it; the fact that you remember it now proves that you saw it, and that it was stored somewhere in your brain. But part of you labeled it insignificant.

This, by the bye, is one of the things you must work on if you want to avoid another sweet-guy-goes-bad situation.

In the old days, denial came in the form of "Oh, that tiger looks old and sick! We need the water so I'm going down anyway.""

Nowadays it's, "Aw, he only said that because he was drunk!"

That's denial. Yeah, you do it too—but only when the truth is to painful to look at in the face.

You thought like that when you saw signs of a horsey butt early on mainly because you were influenced by the powerful chemistry of attraction—hormonal (which opens new doors in how your brain can slam doors, believing it's a survival issue). Add to that influence all those stories you were told or have read about "true love," and "true love" music, movies, blogs. They may be entertaining stories, but they are fairy tales. No more true than cartoon stories.

Should you two years down the road look in on the same couple you've read about having a happy ending, what will you see? Unless they both of them are heavily equipped with heathy relationship skills, and problem-solving skills, and patience, their relationship will have become very like yours. Good examples of this brain wiring are easier seen in the rat or bird when they don't see the cat or snake moving in; it's because it moves in very slowly.

For the rat (and the weight-gainer) small changes slip through the brain's mental screen. In some cases, they (and we) dismiss those we see, even when they are life-threatening. On the other hand, if we noted every little change around us, we might starve to death from lack of fresh meant, or just go mad because we were so distracted. (If every tiniest thing was attended to we'd see a lot of cat and snake skeletons—having died of hunger.)

Your brain tends to retain an instilled memory. The instilled, engraved memory is created when emotion is attached to the event. If you are startled, and you are a rat, you will note precisely where that cat is at the moment.

You were flooded with emotion early on in your relationship; who he was then was heavily engraved. Most of you probably had it engraved as deeply as it would be with a branding iron—all because of the throng of powerful emotions and biochemicals flying through your bloodstream day and night.

The more emotion, the deeper the impression go—and the deeper it will stay. That early mental picture tends to stick. If you had formed a new picture of your guy with every tiny change, or if you blatantly kept score, posted on a scoreboard how many times he acted ugly or said ugly things, your brain wouldn't have energy or space available to do all the other things required for survival. But—you wouldn't be in this situation you're in now.

This explains how your lover can come home irritable, and you, impressed with his better state, say to yourself: "Oh, it's just the stress of work, it's only temporary, no big deal; if I'm sweet as Belle was to Beast, this ugly suit will fall off."

You excuse, then dismiss, those early little bits of ugliness that, if you were tuned (had been taught) to take seriously negative behavior, your situation would be different—even if your loving self stayed the same.

"Sit down baby, poor baby! You must have had an awful day! You don't really think I'm a crazy b--. Here, let me massage your neck, darlin'."

Note what you're thinking then, "If I'm sweet enough, he'll get better! He'll see how valuable I am and love me more."

Say this happens two or three times a week for a while, until one day you realize that he's on vacation and has had fun all day, so being ugly can't be for all the old reasons. But by then, you may have been ground down enough you don't think of that.

This is how the brain works. In animals too. The more you get used to something, the more trivial it will appear. Being nice all the time loses its flavor to those it's meant to benefit.

Most drinkers's women continue that thinking for those five to twenty years—while he grows big hairy ears, big ugly nose, and fangs.

This didn't happen because you're stupid.

It happened because of your special wiring got twisted up with the ugly part of his disorder. If either piece of that formula is missing, we don't get a drinker's woman.

The solution is to dig for and get new information. Rewire that part of your brain. It's easier than you think.

And cut yourself some slack now that you understand what's really been going on.

It can be hard to pinpoint when a his changes first appeared, but it's easy to imprint a new mental picture in your subconscious, one that clearly shows his changes. Comfort your Inner Child with assurances that she's going to have more fun as you Thought-Switch, seeing only him as he has become.

Think about what you're seeing and stir up some emotion about how he's ugly, as you remember that he has cheated you, maybe cheated on you, and developed a mean mouth.

Step back and look at what he promised: love and care. Then open your eyes and see clearly what he's doing now. Be outraged!

Being angry is not a sin. It can flush away your innate system of condemning yourself. While you may dread it, getting mad is good, good for you. It changes your chemistry—and that changes the way your brain thinks. It's dandy to get mad!

Start thinking things like, "Just who does he think he is by criticizing you, raging at you, controlling you (and if not physically, then certainly he has been mentally and emotionally beating you into submission). And you have become stuck in staying anxious about not being perfect enough to meet the standards of a Horse's Butt!

Slam that Today Picture up beside a mental picture of the guy you fell in love with. Aw-w, he was so sweet, so romantic. Smiling, cute, fun, focused on you, treasuring you, wanting to please you. Okay Hold It! Click and Save. What happened? I suggest you go into any stash of photos of the two of you early on, or even just of him.

Once you have these pictures clearly in mind, pull up another mental picture to paste up beside them. This one of him during his last temper tantrum. And add snapshots to this collection as soon as you glimpse or remember them. How about one that's just as he may be at the moment: sitting on the couch, beer in one hand, channel-changer in the other hand, and recall the ugly words recently rolling out of his mouth.

This mental maneuver will replace your pain with reality. You are still in love with something that doesn't exist anymore. Allow the emotion stirred by this exercise to grow strong enough to fully imprint the new picture, reality.

You once had an ice-cream cone, but it's melted.

Now you see it; now you don't.

Your caring, loving self has automatically categorized all his glitches as "temporary," believing the fairy tales that float around that (if *you* just did the right thing) *he'd* go back to being his sweet, cute, fun self.

But you have stayed sweet—at least sweeter than anyone else in the world could have stayed—and he hasn't reverted to prince, has he?

The purpose of this book is to tell you that it's not likely ever to happen. If that's the case, you can see clearer how to make your own life better.

I Remember . . . *My last (and most painful) breakup.*
I was moving out, packing a photo album the two of us had put together early in our relationship; a handful of pictures slid out. I opened the album to replace them and there, on the first pages, I saw him—so cute, so sweet. My heart wailed with the pain of it. I had loved him so much. Memories of how cute and sweet he was brought a sharp pang of loss—grief for those sweet days. In an instant doubts flooded me: was I making a terrible mistake by leaving? Such a cute and fun guy.

Feeling awful, I replaced the fallen pictures and another photo slipped out. I picked it up and began to automatically throw it away. It was a terrible picture of him, taken actually only a week or two earlier. The picture had been so ugly that I hadn't pasted it in the album, intending to toss it. Which turned out to be great good fortune.

A startling feeling now—confidence—and the grief and self-doubt evaporated instantly upon looking at this picture.

What a difference between this picture and the first one! So sweet, then Really Uhhhgg-ly. Seven years after the first picture, he was fat, seedy, his belly hanging over his belt. He looked out at me, his face sarcastic, arrogant, a sneer as he stared out at me, just as he had done that day when I took this picture. His body language clearly conveyed that he not only didn't care about me anymore, not about my happiness or my love for him, but clearly reflected the way he felt about me now.

As to my being unhappy now, he told me frequently that my unhappiness was of my own making. He said I made myself miserable. Well, I surely was that—miserable. But I had learned enough to know that it wasn't all me.

The grief and loneliness I was feeling was focused on how wonderful he was (no—how wonderful he was back then).

Then—Flash!—I got a full dose of reality, of his massive change from that old picture to this last picture: I doubted many would believe they were both the same man.

As the reality of what I was seeing hit home, I set the "now" picture aside to stick up on my new refrigerator. I realized the blast of relief reality I'd just received.

I needed that picture I taped to my new refrigerator in my new home. I used it to relieve that terrible grief and self-doubt that continued to rise up frequently until the fantasy, the "wish" that he was still the guy from the past, morphed to a realistic acceptance of the present reality.

Whenever I became aware that I was doing "it" again— grieving for something that no longer existed—I took myself to the refrigerator—not to munch (most of the time), but to stand there and take in the "now" picture.

Each time I looked at it, any pain I was feeling vanished— poof! In its place came a flood of relief—with a tinge of giddiness—that I was free of what had become a painful mess.

Over the next few months, every time I started wallowing, or feeling blue, I went to the refrigerator and got a flash of reality. I am quite sure I did that, not because I'm so smart, but because of the instant rush of relief that followed registering the new reality. That "now" photo showed me of what I had really lost.

Pain. Misery. Ugliness. I could clearly see that what I had been grieving for was like a fantasy! I was grieving for something that didn't even exist anymore, working so hard to transform what I saw in the now back into the cute, fun him.

*When I began to see the reality of what he had become, it wiped away the pain and self-doubt. The picture trick worked **every** time I got into that self-doubting mindset. I set out to imprint reality, that what I had lost wasn't the sweet guy.*

That guy had been gone for a long time.

In fact, what I had lost had turned into something I didn't want back.

Today, 20-something years later, when I think of that man, I can only envision the "now" picture. And every single time this occurs, after 20 years, I still get a rush of joy just to be free!

Other Reasons You "Missed It"

We both know that you didn't fall in love with a Horse's Butt, and that you didn't stupidly "miss it."

You saw, you interpreted what you saw in a positive way, which is a beautiful quality, one I'm sure the angels sing over—giving people the benefit of the doubt.

When you met this man, your hormones and your romantic nature decided that he was or could be The One.

You operated on a tremendously strong drive wired into women (perhaps a dirty trick, bringing to mind the curse I've read in the Book of Genesis, a curse that fell on all women for the poor judgement of one).

What can a girl do about this tendency?

One answer is to never, ever again surrender to the strong romantic blur that occurs when a potential "mate" comes into view. Enjoy the feeling, if you can do so without projecting the wedding. Don't go there. And don't allow those chemicals to affect your judgement and clarity of vision.

Remember: A psychopath can be charming right up until he stabs you in the back.

Psych Note: You need not fear that happening to you once you learn how to spot a psychopath or a narcissist. Hold back your excitement chemistry while you take a sufficient amount of time to check him out for self-centeredness, for trying too hard, usually for bragging, and especially for the way he talks about other people—most obvious at first when it's about people you don't know, such as other drivers on the road, or a young person walking down the street.

Holding down the rush of excited chemistry early on, you

definitely are smart enough to soon pick up on when he judges other people negatively and doesn't have much feeling for people, especially not for their pain or unhappiness. You look for if they tend to criticize, put down others, or—importantly—pick of signals of a wandering eye. ("Looking" at another female while he's with you is a reliable signal of the wandering eye. That particular disorder never, ever goes away. It will linger long after he's lost all the equipment to do anything about it.)

You can even test a guy by tossing out comments occasionally--something like you feel compassion for the homeless, or poor, or disadvantaged. *If he puts them down, or tries to correct you to quit feeling for them, it he says negative things about them, you have a self-centered narcissist on your hands (at best). Time to Move Along.*
The longer you stay near him, the longer he has to sink his hook into you. Many of these dangerous creatures have excellent skills for hooking and ripping apart caring women. Using them up, and moving on—telling them they're leaving because they've become ugly and grouchy.
A narcissist isn't necessarily a psychopath, but the psychopath is almost always narcissistic.
Living with a narcissist who never drinks can be almost as bad as living with a man who drinks too much. (Of course, many of them are or become narcissists too.)
Of course, pay very close attention to how he drinks. Most over-drinkers consider themselves "a social drinker." Watch out for the phrase. It's not scripture here, just common signals of an unworthy potential partner.

It's hard to let go of that dream, the hope, that romance will eventually win out, that we'll all live happily ever after. The same novels and movies and stories and music that imprinted a lot of your beliefs about love continue to pummel you with their erroneous imaginations. These ideas are hard to shed; they've been with us for a long time, they form part of your narrow vision of a new lover. Believing in Santa Claus is not as dangerous as believing in Prince Charming. Believing he's your own Prince overshadows your judgement of everything he does. Right up until his fangs are fully grown out.
But believe me on this extremely important adjustment that you absolutely must make (or suffer terrible emotional wounds

for the rest of your life): The smallest sign of an ugly person is meaningful!

It gives you a glimpse of how bad this person can become—and then think of how miserable it will be to live with such a mean-hearted, self-centered, negative man. Who very likely will become an over-drinker. You'll want to "alibi" the bad behavior you see, "give him he benefit of the doubt." Don't! A person who has none of those tendencies won't say or do the things you're watching for.

Pay attention with a new guy.
Back off when you see the signals!

And hold back your romantic excitement over a new guy until you've carefully examined how he thinks about and treats others. Consider: How can the real Prince Charming get through to you if you're all wrapped up with an unworthy man, trying to pull your fantasy prince out of a beast.

FACT
A potential lover cannot (and will not) fake a bad behavior. That means that if you see it, especially early on, you can believe it's really him!

The special kind of partner that you are doesn't need to ever feel so desperate for someone to care for her as to take in or accept anything less than a proven good heart, and established good behavior.

Only a good heart can match your own and even come near a promise of real love.

The stakes are high in this new lesson. If a bad sign arises early in a relationship, you now err on the side of safety and mark it down as a signal of what's really inside him.

And the slightest bad behavior you see in him signals what your future will almost certainly contain with that man.

Mistaken Ideas

Let's examine three major mistaken ideas you and most other little girls have grown up with. These mistaken ideas are responsible for the bulk of your wearing blinders where a new man is concerned. They have been imbedded in your bedtime stories, cartoons you watched, comic books, movies you saw, books you read, and TV shows. And you have been told and believed that they are just fairy tales. BUT—they have silently been shaping your attitudes.

Mistake Number 1: Failing to connect a bad behavior to having no love. At the same time, you latch onto the least nice thing he does and use it to build your fairy castle, mistaking a few nice things for love. Furthermore, you must understand that people can have both qualities; what you're guarding against is nastiness, heartless, selfish thinking and behavior. Those tell you that you are looking at a loser.

Reality: Love is not a feeling; it's living action. Love isn't what someone feels or says, though if it's real they will feel and say these things. Feeling good and saying love things do not prove love. On the other hand, ugly attitudes, when spotted do prove the absence of love, likely of the ability to love—unselfish love. But it's what he does that speaks love , and not just a few examples when the romance is new.

The tenderness and caring and unselfishness and lack of criticizing anyone—when those last for any length of time—even a month—you've probably got a winner on your hands. Of course, as you know, a winner can become a loser over time, no matter how carefully you check him out in advance. Still, look for the demonstration of the right thinking in him before surrendering your trust to him.

Mistake Number 2: Believing the fairy tales are real, that they reflect real life, fairy tales such as stories about how love could heal a man of ugliness, and that doing *the right thing* will make him change.

Reality: Any change in another person is a *him*-thing; it's **never** going to be a you-thing—something you create.

Some people say that a man changed for love of his woman, but that was still a him-thing. Knowing what's wrong with him before you open your heart is vitally important.

Once you open your heart, it slaps the blinders on.

3. Mistake: The idea of what love *is* has been greatly distorted—with things like the idea that love can happen immediately. Love doesn't. Attraction, extremely strong attraction, happens fast, immediately. But not love. Love grows like a plant from a seed, not exploding like fireworks.

Reality: You can determine real love by first learning what it absolutely isn't: Hurting your partner—physically or emotionally—does not arise from love. Calling someone bad names, mocking them, bullying, controlling—all have nothing of love in them. In love, those things cannot exist.

A Horse's Butt in Nice Guy Clothing
You are not stupid! Here's proof: What happens mentally when you run into a new person with ugly behavior?

Right. You Move Along. No exciting romantic feelings appear.

And now you can see that you would never have fallen in love with this man as he is today.

(Note: A few of you may have had the idea that a guy can be bad to other people, but he won't be to you. Maybe you see a tough guy as a protector. Oh, my dear, that's so-o-o wrong.

(The sure way to spot a man well on the way to Horse's Butt is noticing the way he treats (and talks about) other people. If he's critical, puts others down as if he is far superior, or shows in any ay that others's feelings are meaningless to him, you can be sure he's not your Prince. He's a Beast in sheep's clothing. If he often points out others imperfections, he needs to go. That mindset is based on deep-seated emotional problems and you and your love cannot heal him.

(At the same time, if a guy (even a less attractive guy) frequently points the good qualities in people, you've got a keeper. This man has the potential to be wonderful life mate.)

Some Bad News
One of the most difficult truths of this book is that you probably will never get back that great guy you fell for. Even if he finds recovery and sticks with it (which, you've already learned, is a desperately slim chance that will almost surely take years for his brain and personality to begin to rise above the damaged thinking and behavior he has developed. (How hard is it for you to break a habit? Well, brain reshaping is stronger than habit.)

Point to Implant: After the five to twenty more years it will take for him to become the stereotype drunkard, this guy may be diagnosed as needing help. Then, if he submits, the weeks or months it takes for him to get rooted in the required recovery lifestyle, you'll still have to wait more months, even years for him to get back just parts of who he used to be. If he ever does that at all. So here's your question for the day: How old will you be then?

Reality is your "today" photo, his today actions!

So—What Can You Do about Horsey-Butt Behavior?
Very little, and likely, nothing. The saddest part of this story is that the so-called Prince was born with a genetic glitch that would make it easy for him to become an over-drinker, and possibly warp his personality in other negative ways. His susceptibility to a drinking problem could come from a crossed wire in his brain, genetic or otherwise; maybe he's missing some cells in a key organ like his liver or pancreas, even his brain, that make it impossible for his body to process alcohol as well as others do. Try to keep this in mind—not to alter your decisions about whether you can live this way, but to help you avoid hating him. Hatred is the poison that kills the one who uses it.

What was likely a snafu in his genetic structure preordained a horrible fate for him—and for those close to him.

Another very important question: What do you think you can do about his genetic structure?

Nothing? Right.

That's sad. But no matter how sad the early lives of many foul people were, other people aren't required to just sit there and take it because they feel sorry for them. Or to somehow make up for their earlier misery.

With a genetic glitch, you can't do anything to fix it. His body and brain from birth were set to not adequately process alcohol, meaning that if he drank much at all, it would do him great damage. But you cannot change any part of that. And you cannot erase the damage. In other words, there is nothing you can do or say to fix his problem.

It's nice to replace hate or bitterness with pity, but don't buy into his wish that you bear his burdens. Pity does not require spending the rest of your life trying to fix something that only he can fix. If he wants you to do it, or says he can't do it without you, he's fooling himself. He's good at that.

Just don't let him fool you into believing him. It can be easy to fall into that trap because most of you need love so badly by then it's like turning down a cookie when you're starved. But you do turn down this "bribe" of shallow love, if it isn't just fake by now. That because this tempting cookie is attached to the rest of the bag.

* * *

Rethinking Your "Now" Reality

Does it make any sense to argue with someone who has an impaired brain?   Yes   No

Especially once he's taken even one drink?

And does it make sense to argue with someone who is willing to hurt you (at least emotionally) in order to win?   Yes   No

Arguing with him about anything is a waste of your energy and spirit, energy and spirit you could be using to do something positive in your own life.

Realize that In taking care of yourself, you take care of the whole world. If you are not okay, you can't do much for anyone else. You owe it to the world who can be helped by you, and to your God, to take care of yourself and not waste your spirit.

Because of alcohol's rapid effect on his brain, once he takes a single drink his reason begins to slip. His judgement center is already numbing-down. Besides, even if you should win the lottery—I mean win the argument, it won't change anything. At least, not for long. Has it ever?

The moment you tell him you want to discuss something serious, the first thing he wants to do is get a drink. But you can now see that after the first swallow, your attempts to resolve problems are almost certainly doomed. Make your decision now to save that energy. Use it to do something fun.

Once he's had even a swallow of alcohol, you may as well spend your energy hollering down a well. (Which is preferable because a well won't call you ugly names and bring up every mistake you've ever made.)

What? Did I hear you say you you're going to Move Along and go do something fun?

Maybe even get a life?

Psych Note: Another brain area that when affected makes it

> impossible to get through to him once he even starts to drink is his reward center. That's the part of the brain that notes when something is rewarding and sends out messages to other parts of the brain to look for more of whatever brought the good feeling.
>
> His first drink is already touching his brain cells the way he wants it to and that is extremely rewarding. It's the feeling he longs for. The reward center is an extremely loud and powerful brain sector. It shouts in all of us things like, "I want that chocolate!" "I want those shoes!" "I want that drink!"

That "desire" comes from its memory of the pleasant feeling it gets when he gets the wanted item. Your reward center remembers *everything* that you enjoy and how you obtain it.

When it wants that feeling, believes it needs that feeling, it prods the rest of the brain to fire up his entire body to go fetch.

The very first dose of alcohol immediately begins changing his brain chemistry. The specific chemistry change feels very good to him. Sometimes it's because a body doesn't produce enough of the feel-good chemical on its own. But he quickly loses whatever ability to achieve the good feeling in any other way, only the alcohol will do. Part of the reason is because its action is so rapid.

No matter how many times you tell him that drinking is not good for him, no matter how many times you get him to actually agree with you, when he begins to feel the stress, the need, his reward center shouts you down, and negates his good intentions. And the first drink feels so good that it makes him want another.

He is affected from the very first drink and that is why you can trust your senses to recognize it, even if he's had only one. All his verbal denial and flaring up at you won't change the changes in him that alcohol has already begun making.

By the time his drinks don't make him feel so good anymore, his judgement center is pretty much shot, so instead of making a good decision, he doesn't see any reason to stop drinking. His survival instincts also shut down, pretty much all of it except the part that thinks that he must have alcohol for his survival. He can't admit that to himself, much less to anyone else.

* * *

Whatcha Got in Your Bag of Tricks So Far?

With the tricks you've begun learning, you already have a reliable bag of simple tactics that can change-modify, if not erase, almost every one of your common ugly situations.

You now know tricks that
- let you sidestep most of his chaos,
- easily to avoid or duck out of arguments,
- ignore his mean words,
- and if an argument flashes before you remember to use your tricks, *you can still pull them out and use them* at that time—*and they will still work*.
- You also know a trick or two to get yourself back into a peaceful balance.
- You also have the basic part of the trick to stop berating yourself when you're not perfect; you just talking back to the mean voice, telling it some of the good things do and the good things you do.

And No, He Can't (Won't) See what He's Doing to You
Part of you may still believe that he'd change if only he would only see how bad he's hurting you. In fact, he may have lied to himself so much already that he feels good when you suffer because he blames you for much of his misery.

The same brain damages that rob him of his sound reason and his ability to maintain good control over his negative emotions and behaviors also blind him to how his behavior affects others.

This is why you are going to let go of your focus on making sure he knows. Even should he get a glimpse of it, he may already be incapable of doing much about it.

Changing once he sees how his behavior is affecting you only works in the Very Early Stage. If he has become so bad you are reading this book, he's wa-ay beyond the Early Stage.
And beyond being able to change for your sake.

Trying to figure out how to get him to see what he's doing to you can eat you alive. (Women tend to believe this should be a successful tactic because we are actually wired to be very sensitive to the emotional condition and needs of others. Men aren't. Any of that ability they have, they've probably had to work for. Indeed, men don't even have that hunk of brain.

You've probably exerted yourself trying to follow his logic, trying to understand. The problem is that following his logic requires that you follow the logic and reasoning of a sane man. The result is that you come away feeling like you're the one screwed up, but you're not! It's him.

Trying to understand *why* he says the things he says is more wasted energy. Arguing with the things he says a out you is hard to resist, but it's a total waste. And it likely is playing right into his scheme to get away and blame you. *The reason, the only reason, he says the things he says against you is that he has noticed the effect they have and he wants to create that effect now.*

As to getting through to him, you can do that, even point out negatives, but it must be done at special times and in a special way. Best you can, leave off trying to get through until you get to that section of this book.

When you're upset, he can use that to convince you that you're the one who's crazy. But being upset is the normal response to his abnormal thinking and behavior. If you buy into what he makes of your being upset, he will unstoppably go on to blame you for whatever he decides to do next. He can blame you, escape the guilt, and go do something fun, and what happens to you? You become more despondent, less sure of yourself, and start to feel inadequate and trapped. Yeah, it's a boon for him when he can get you upset.

Adding value to this experience he now can throw your incident of upset back at you, over and over, for the rest of your natural life.

Folding, flinching, answering back to whatever he says, especially to defend yourself, all simply trigger his now fueled-up reflex to come back at you, and it will always be meaner than what he said before. His load of frustration and rage is looking for somewhere to blow out.

Why bother defending yourself to a man who is mentally slipping down the drain. And has it ever worked? So stop trying.

To live around what he is becoming, to save yourself, you must remind yourself constantly that he uses words, accusations, criticisms, potshots, whatever comes to him at the time, to hurt you, upset you. All this to shut you up when you say something that he doesn't like, such as telling him he's drinking too much.

Even if he actually believes you're crazy, arguing with his stupid statement can make you look crazier. Let Go! Move Along! With or without Stretchy Lip.

Get this: At the peak of an argument, using his words for their effect on you, upsetting you, hurting you, seeing you in tears, he can throw up his hands dramatically and exclaim, "Oh, my god, I've got to get out of here!"

Slam!

Having gotten you upset enough to blame his leaving on you, he goes to drink and play without guilt. He tells himself (and others) that he deserves a drink because he's got a crazy wife!

You have an Inner Actress. Remember her? (She's the one who used to play with her dolls, and now she's the one whosmiles and says, "Fine," when others ask how you are.) Since showing you are upset digs a hole for you to fall into, call out your lovely Inner Actress when he starts his stuff.

Get this: You don't have to be unruffled, just appear to be. Your Inner actress can pull this off, believe it. Your favorite actresses don't have to actually be whatever they are playing—they are acting! And you can do the same thing.

Pretend his words don't bother you. You can even appear distracted, as if thinking about something, and asking him, "What did you just say? I'm sorry—I missed it."

You'll discover how easy it is to put a crimp in his act.

Bonus: Slipping into your Inner Actress is great fun!

Psych Note: Brain changes causes personality change. Brain changes do not snap back to their former shape. Not in him, and also not in you. The wounds you receive when you listen to and believe his words leave a scar. Emotional scars pile up to create walls that block out all the good in life, strangely staying wide open to whatever he says.

You are enacting something you may have learned as a very small child—to listen to someone's reason for being angry or punishing you, or withdrawing approval or love. You learned to listen carefully so you could correct whatever it was and finally earn love.

Accepting now that his brain is getting whacky allows you to absorb that it doesn't matter whether he really believes the mean things he says.

What's important is that your feelings are less important to him that whatever he's trying to accomplish with his mean words. His focus is on getting what he wants; he is truly incapable of really knowing, or caring, that his words are hurting you.

When he is mean to you, or leaves you by yourself, or says mean things about you, when he threatens to get another woman, he's not saying those things out of love.

Don't fool yourself about this.

Whatever he feels, it's no longer love. He may need you; he may want you in case he needs you to do something; but he doesn't love you. Love is gentle, love is kind, love is merciful, love is not ugly and it doesn't try to hurt its object. Some of you are familiar with a letter from a man named Paul to a group of people in Corinth where he sets forth so beautifully what love really is.

* * *

A Tad More Bad News

If he continues to drink anything—even in small amounts—His Horse's-Butt personality eventually takes him over.

In addition, his occasional flashes of Mr. Sweet Guy that used to confuse you, won't much longer; that's because Mr. Sweet Guy also goes totally extinct. Time for another new trick. The Refuse to Answer a Horse's Butt Trick:

Do you remember the game of Pin the Tail on the Donkey? I'm old, and you're not as old as me, so you may not have played that game when you were a child. It's a game where grownups pin up a poster with a huge picture of a goofy looking donkey—with a big rear end, but no tail. They the grownups blindfold the children, one by one, hand them a paper donkey's tale with a tack or tape on the top end, spin the child around and point them toward the poster. The blindfolded child then places the tale where he believes it should go. And everybody laughs and laughs because it's usually on his nose—or worse. The child who comes closest to the right spot wins a prize.

Now that you know what the game is, get a mental picture of

what that cartoon donkey looks like, looking back at you over his shoulder and over his huge behind. This is the picture that will work a miracle: When he begins any form of rant, pull up a mental picture of that dopey, grinning, big-butted donkey, and see if you can take anything he says seriously.

You use this trick to avoid arguing back against any negative thing he says about you.

This mental trick wipes out the effect of his harangue, and will usually tickle your funny bone. You may even discover a real smile on your own face when you use this trick.

The Refuse-to-Answer-a-Horse's-Butt Trick

1. . **Catch** your rising tension!

2. **Picture** the dopey-donkey with a huge but and your mate's head.

3. Place the mental picture directly over where he is sitting or standing.

4. **Stretch 'Em** and Move Along.

5. Keep your focus on Move Along. This trick shuts the mental door that lets new junk in. You can only focus on one thing at a time.

Now for a mental run-through, a practice:
Picture him right now saying something mean, then pop out your mental donkey poster and picture that face as his, that pose as his. Do that two or three times, or until it starts feeling comfortable, fun.

Beware the Jabberwocky
(a mythical beast created by Lewis Carroll, author of "Alice's Adventures in Wonderland)

As you begin taking care of yourself emotionally, you can count on this: He's going to try harder. He'll egg you on, especially repeating everything he has *ever* found to upset you.

But you are forewarned; expect his tricks, trying to force you into one of your old responses so he can "Slam!" and be gone.

You simply repeat any or all of your tricks, which keeps your attention there instead of straining to hear what he says. Stay firm. Each time, Stretch 'Em, Clamp 'Em, and Move Along!

Once he succeeds in upsetting you, he wins, at least in his own mind—but of course not in yours. When he "wins" you just get back on working through your bag of tricks.

You know not to beat yourself up for collapsing; it will take some time before you lose all fear of his threats of withdrawing love. Now you know there's precious little of it, if any at all. All you need do is Move Along and think how you can do your trick even better next time.

If you get upset or if you don't, it's going to end as it usually ends: He will work himself into a state, then blow up, all the while blaming you for causing it with all your imperfections, and then he will storm out to go get drunk. Which was what he was wanting all along.

Slam! Take a moment to savor the silence.

The Refuse to Answer a Horse's Butt Trick Example

1. If he doesn't slam out, pull out your Oscar-Award-Winning Inner Actress and act the part you used to play naturally: Sweet. "Aw baby—Let me get you a beer and you can just relax."

He'll either leave without winning, Slam! or he'll shut down due to the surprise effect. Repeat your intention of getting him the cold beer, stirring that cold beer desire in him. This will likely sidetrack him from making many more nasty comments .

* * *

Oh! More Things to Know About "Recovery" (And Why Treatment Isn't Necessarily the Answer)

Established beyond any doubt is that an over-drinker is sure to continue getting worse so long as he continues to consume any form of alcohol. With every drink he takes, the cellular damage worsens. It continues to destroy what's left from last time—not only in his brain but also the rest of his body. Damage is piling up in the very organs he needs to process (break down) the alcohol in his blood.

Now his increasing loss of judgement and increasingly muddled thinking guarantee that the one drink will set off his desire for more.

Can you do anything about that? No. And has any scheme you've ever dreamed up done the trick? No. That's why you're here now.

Have you tried to fix it before?

And how did that work?

Most women believe that a drinker's wanting to change is the key to actually changing, but that's not totally correct. Almost every day of an over-drinker's life, he thinks about easing off, cutting down, even quitting. Most of those times, he truly wants to, yet it doesn't work, so wanting to can't be the key.

Has he ever told you that he wants to stop and you believed that he truly meant it. Well, he probably did. He just wasn't ready to do all the things he must do in order to make that happen.

In fact, right now he doesn't even know all the things he must do in order to make that happen. So when he promises, he has no idea what he's promising. Thus, his promise is doomed to be broken.

You know in advance how slim are his chances of quitting and then staying quit, so you be sympathetic if you wish; you know that even if he stops, he'll go back to it. The only question will be when. But you're prepared for that. Now you won't be emotionally shattered when he starts up again.

Don't pay any heed to anyone who slams you with the "negative thinking" angle in regard to this trick. It is not negative thinking to plan for earthquakes or hurricanes so you're ready should one come. You're not being negative when you expect that unsafe sex will get you infected, that cigarettes will fatally damage your heart and lungs. Tell just that to any critics, and remember it yourself.

Your fact of life: You can't make this man drink any more than you can make him stop! *When* (not *if*) he starts up again, he will try every trick in the book to get your goat so he can blame his falling back on you! Be ready.

When it comes: Stretchy Lip him, Move Along, and in this case—leave the area. Find a way to go do something fun.

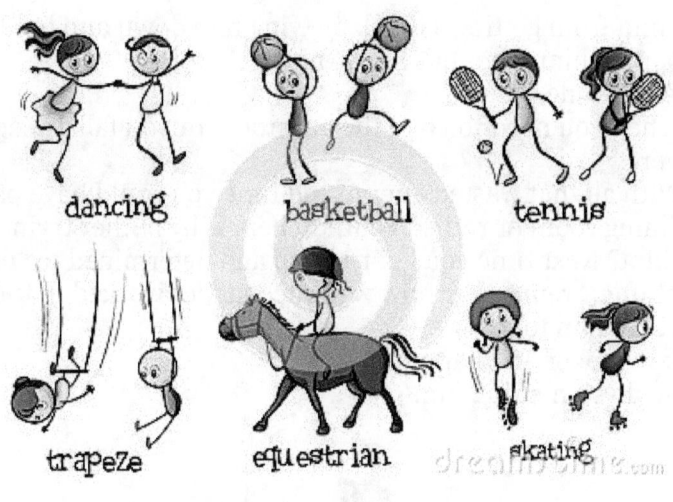

dancing basketball tennis
trapeze equestrian skating

* * *

A man committed to quitting and who is taught how to catch his own tension and use his own tricks will not drink even if you demand it! To get straight and stay straight, the drinker must learn, accept fully that it's the first drink that flips on the craving.

But no one can teach him that and everything else he will need to know except other men who have experienced it and learned how to win. Blaming you is a grand manipulation that he has mastered; it puts him in control. It means nothing that you are left in lonely misery. All that matters is getting what he wants.

(Note: This non-caring behavior too does not arise out of love. It's ego, some mental disorder, or just plain meanness.)

Nothing you can do will prevent him from drinking once he takes a mind to. (This is an experience you've no doubt already had—trying to keep him from drinking when he intends to.) Indeed, you place yourself in harm's way when you try. (And you probably felt like a failure when your attempts didn't work.) In the Early Stages, you may postpone his getting a drink. But even in the Early Stage, it won't be postponed for long.

Time for you to simply relax that part of your mind.

He will find a way to drink when he wants to. Over-drinkers can get booze in treatment! In the hospital. In a mental lock-up, even in jail and prison! In the desert, in the Arctic. You can only keep him from getting a drink by tying him down and holding a weapon on him. That has been known to work.

For a while.

When you need to go to the bathroom or you fall asleep, it's all over.

With all that wasted energy and time you could have painted the dining room or retiled your kitchen. Why bother trying to stop him? Next time you get riled up and determined to "do something," remember how well such tactics worked in the past.

Leave him to it.

Live longer and happier.

Go do something fun.

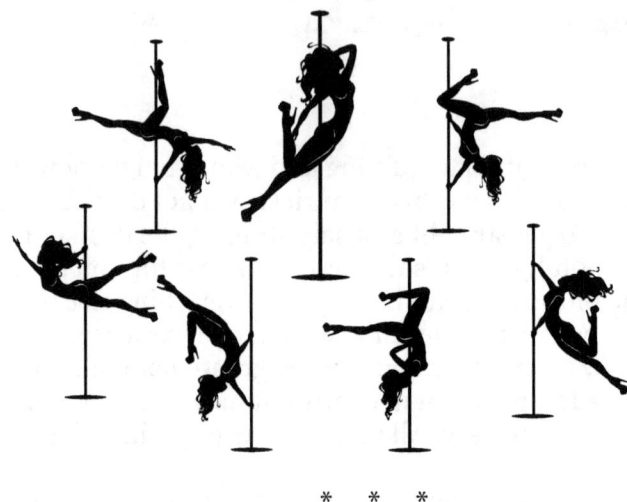

* * *

The stress he feels when wanting a drink escalates his desire for it. His stressful feelings are the main reason he craves that special feeling—that he only gets from alcohol. The deadener.

Good News: It doesn't take long for most over-drinkers to stop trying to blame a partner who responds in the ways you are learning. Once he realizes his tactics really don't work anymore, which means he must try them several times first, he drops them. Just like the pigeons in cages in my old psych labs: When the corn pellets quit coming when they peck a button, they stop pecking.

More Good News: Rebuilding your self-confidence and self-esteem are the easiest fixes in all of psychotherapy! Some licensed therapists can give you the keys to both in one session.

You can get these fixes far easier than you may think—especially if you don't try to do it alone. A therapist or a group are both excellent tools, also lots of the self-help books that are on the market now. On our website I give you many of the books I've read and think are great. When you find others, let us know! Put them in the blog to share with your sisters! And me.

In thinking about your own healing, recollect that wounds from a ballpeen hammer can't heal as long as the hammer is still pounding away. Nor can you heal up and find that precious self when new jabs keep you off balance.

Still More Good News: Once you shut down some of his stuff and learn how to get out of range of the rest of it, you're going to begin to heal naturally. Should you find it's in your best interest to try staying with him, unless he has ever been violent, I'm all for it. Many women have found they could cope with the drinker using the tactics in this book and any outside help you can get. Trying to stay may be the best road for most of you who, I've found, still carry great fear of misjudging, and love. That's fine; take your time, unless he can be violent.

For some, the tricks here gave them what they needed to stay in their relationship while living a fuller and more satisfying life.

If that's what you want, I wish it for you.

Should you decide, however, that it's best to separate, be sure to pay close attention to Chapter 9, especially about planning carefully, and do not talk about it in advance or threaten it. You do it this way because leaving an over-drinker is most dangerous when you're in process. When he believes you really mean it.

It is not sneaky to hide from a sniper. It is not sneaky to hide from flu bugs in a crowd. It is not sneaky to get a vaccination to avoid illness, or to cure a problem with medication. And it is not sneaky to be very careful and quiet about leaving an over-drinker (or any other man) who has the least tendency to violence!

With him or without him, you will need to take time to heal before you expect much of yourself. If you don't take care of yourself, you will never be able to function to your incredible potential. Once removed from the hammering, you will rapidly begin to heal. That's because of who you really are—who you have always been: a truly good, valuable, wonderful, and spunky human being.

The Over-Drinker Also has a Bag of Tricks!

The over-drinker is so good at his tricks (manipulation), that he destroys himself. Letting him off the hook when he pours out his excuses happens because you didn't know that his only hope of changing is to feel the heat. Intensely. His life depends on feeling the heat. And on his tricks failing to work for him anymore.

Engrave across your brain that each time you let him off the hook, you in fact guarantee that he'll do it again!

If he has no negative consequences to his behavior, or if those consequences are minimal, in his mind it's the same as saying, "All right dear, play nice from now on." Like so much else when dealing with an over-drinker, your initial intentions of kindness meant to make him more compliant end up creating just the opposite of what you intended. When you give him your compassion and mercy and forgiveness and patience, he basks in it. It gets even better when you actually help him clean up the mess he's made. You help him get out of a jam to show you love him (and as a bid for him to love you in return). Yet for most over-drinkers, it turns out that they like and respect you less for being so easy to manipulate!

It is only when he can't escape the pain or the humiliation of his own making that he has even the slightest chance of seeing the light. So what are you really accomplishing when you push yourself, stress yourself, to make him more comfortable with the consequences of his own making—from easing his hangovers to paying his bail bond? And have those precious gifts to him ever brought the love and appreciation you craved. Or the improved behavior you prayed for.

When you lighten his consequences, putting off his having to pay the piper, you prevent his ever being able to suffer enough to finally think about changing.

And it's going to take quite a bit of suffering.

Here are the facts, ma'am: Even if all the problems that he claims make him drink and behave badly actually did, spending your time and energy trying to fix them won't work; it actually rewards him for manipulating you. He learns he can misbehave, have a blast with no sense of responsibility, and others will clean up. Not much incentive there to change anything, is there?

You can't change his childhood, or what it taught him—no matter how much you love him and try to.

No one can love an over-drinker enough to heal what's really wrong with him. That is like trying to love someone so much he'll be cured of cancer.

Only he can fix him. And he must want to be fixed terribly bad, because the cure seems worse than the problem.

Problem is that you have a center that is set on finding a solution. The only solution you have a chance with is leaving him to hurt himself so badly that he wants help, that he begs for help.

Since all your best efforts have failed up to now, let's change off. Let's begin the wonderful and exciting work of healing you. First, we'll work on soothing your urges to fix him. I'm not saying to stop it, to go cold turkey, merely to begin tempering how nice you are. Adjusting your urges is done bit by bit. You can get a head start on this by answering the following questions, and keeping those answers firmly in mind.

Pop Quiz

Why do you believe you need to fix things for him? Make them easier? (Start your answer by being sure to write the first responses that come to mind.)

_____

_____

_____

_____

_____

Take what you come up with here to a trusted friend—or a qualified counselor—and begin work on better understanding this need or drive in you. Enlisting help to change what needs to be changed in yourself. (And self-help books have been proved to be very good resources for personal change.)

Needing appreciation is part of the human wiring; needing it from a specific person—after childhood—can be very destructive. You can want approval, appreciation, even love or admiration from a given individual, but you cannot need it, crave it, demand it, to make it happen.)

There's a difference between preferring something and needing it, or demanding it. When I just prefer something, I'm not distraught and off-balance if I don't get it.

Another question:
How successful have your methods to get what you're seeking been so far?
_____ Very Successful
_____ Not Very Successful
What do you intend to do about that?

_____

_____

For the bad actor to want to change, he *must* suffer for the bad behavior.
I say this emphatically because you are one of those tender spirits. You would never have come to this point if you were otherwise. Unless he desperately wants, begs for, and becomes willing to do whatever is required to change, it's a bust.

You don't do anything to help because he promises to be better. You may choose to help (I advise against it, but you have free will), just don't buy into his promises. As we've seen, he may believe them himself, but he simply isn't able to carry through.

You won't have to create pain for him; he'll do plenty of that if left to himself. Just back off; give him his head—except where it affects your welfare—and refuse to clean up his messes.

You are taming your urge to rush to his rescue. It is difficult; every part of you feels like you "should," that you must help him. Why do you think you think that way?

_____

_____

_____

A big part of you may want to show or prove your love by being there for him—but why? Usually it's so he'll love you in return, maybe enough to stop his "stuff."

Recall that even when you've gone to his rescue in the past, he didn't love you more. At least not for more than a few hours (maybe a few days).

That means it wasn't even real love you got for your trouble.

Doing more for him now, cleaning up his mess, won't earn his love or even his gratitude for long. In a short time he will be criticizing or blaming you again, just as if you hadn't just come to his rescue. The over-drinker is a great example of the saying, "But what have you done for me lately?"

The change you are now beginning will bring you renewed energy, as well as a boost in brain power. Most pleasant of all, you'll probably soon be getting an exhilarating sense of freedom. And little pops of hope or joy.

Your changes, resulting in improved conditions, trigger your subconscious to go for more! This means you really don't have to work very hard at this to succeed—just dabble in it, and your subconscious will pick up on any rewards and start its own engines.

For your physical and mental health, you now focus on doing what's right and good for you. Do this as energetically as you ever have done what's right and good for others.

And one of the best results of this work is your sense of humor begins to return.

You'll know you've become a master when you screw up, and instead of fussing at yourself, you laugh—and then tell someone about it and the two of you laugh together. (Freud said that the ability to laugh at oneself is the greatest sign of good mental health.)

* * *

The Wait 'Til He's Hung-over Trick!

The only way you can get through to his impaired brain now that his denial system is in full bloom is to wait until he's hung-over.

Not only is he suffering great pain and distracted and weakened by it—his defenses are still drunk! His barriers are down and he is more open to suggestions (but not anger or guilt.

He may argue, but if you speak with respect, calmly, simply stating facts—not your feelings!--your points will get in. (Actually, the arguing back at you that you dread? That is the proof that whatever you said has hit its mark. Therefore, don't fear what he'll say; welcome it! Now you know something for sure.)

This hangover trick brings you a gift: You gradually become convinced that his popping off at you is meaningless—and about nothing. Even exploding; you now know it's about him; he needs to blow off steam; you were first in. He aims his venom at you because you're close—not because you really are a bad person. His blowing up is all and only about him. And his payoff is that usually it makes you easy to manipulate.

The Wait for the Hangover Trick

1. Before you speak to him about a behavior, list your reasons for not wanting any more of it. (Only bring up one, a single behavior, at any one talk. You have vastly more impact when you keep it simple; avoid any explanations, no long descriptions. Knowing you'll only be discussing one thing lifts the pressure. Keep it short! The shorter your speech, the deeper in it goes. Don't give him enough time to close you down.

2. Tell him, in a calm voice, the behavior you want him to change, and just how you want it to change. Then hush. Clamp 'Em. Leave the area before he has time to come back at you.

3. If he wants to talk about it, count to three, then you can tell him the kind of thing you'd rather see him do. Don't go into the bad behavior anymore—if you can avoid it because, whether he reacts with anger or guilt, both emotions will block thinking about change. Plus, every word you utter gives him a possible opening to protest or argue. Example of a clear, *very short* statement of what you'd like to see: "I'd really like to see you coming home without puking in the hall."

> **Psych Note:** Research shows that you get far better responses when discussing anything touchy when you keep the focus on a single bad behavior. Do not add anything else (while you've got his attention! It will be tempting. Fight temptation!)
>
> Especially avoid talking about "drinking"—because of the guilt-to-anger reaction he will certainly resort to. Then all your hard work goes down the toilet.

Deliver your statement and Move Along.
When hung-over, his defenses are still drunk; his body (and

mind) are greatly weakened. Tip-toe around arousing his defenses, because guilt will energize him, scrambling for a way to blame it all on you.

Put thought into this trick because it can be an extremely effective one. Not for stopping the drinking, but for changing a single behavior.

Do your best to keep this talk to just one behavior.

And keep it short. Keep it simple. (That's why you plan it in advance, and practice it several times too.)

Do not be drawn into explaining. Or arguing.

You carefully avoid putting any blame on him; this avoids arousing his defenses. That's best done by using "I" statements, "I have been terribly unhappy since you began _____ (fill in the blank). I want you to stop doing that."

(Do not add a threat! For example, don't say, "If you don't do what I ask, I'll leave.") Keep any form of threats out of these conversations.

Threats can only inflame him, which blows away what you were trying to accomplish. And you do the talking. Do not ask for him to respond. Just say it, and quickly Move Along.

You leave the idea and the sound of your voice ringing in his ears.

Clamping jaws and Move Along help keep it short. You do this, not because you're a wimp, but because argument and blame are his forte! He's a master. Recognize that and Move Along.

The next step is easy: Just wait. He will respond—one way or another. You need say no more. Not one word. The rage that can stir up has the power to diminish what you said. The rage can make him think that you deserve to suffer.

On the other hand, he may come to you later, penitent. Don't buy it. Say gently, "If you agree, just show me."

And Move Along again.

Most likely, when he comes out, he'll have some nasty words to throw at you. He may come to you to argue about it. Just refuse. Move Along—no Stretchy-Lip.

Expecting this bad behavior prevents your Tiny Surprise and Brain Freeze

What you're doing is avoiding falling into those argument tricks he's so good at. If he vows to change, tell him that he must show it, demonstrate that he's telling the truth, that then you can believe him. The power of this trick makes it well worth waiting for the next hangover, holding your tongue for when it will do some good. (One positive thing about his drinking: We know the next hangover is coming, you won't have to wait long to speak.)

Once his defenses are aroused (by blame or criticism or disrespect—although he deserves all that and more) his ears slam shut. Not only is further comment from you a waste, he wants it because it stirs up the flame of rage he's wanting to dump, and his mean mouth flies open.

To the best of your ability at the moment, work up some respect for him before you go for "the talk." Even if you have to go wa-ay back and see him as the sweet guy he once was to set your mind. Experience has shown that just a little bit of respect has made all the difference in the effectiveness of this trick. (He has come to think so badly of himself as to be utterly ego-deflated—no matter how loudly he crows. Anything that gives him the sense that you have even a *little* respect for him makes it easier to avoid his anger or arouse his defenses. As much.

Alternate Wait for the Hangover Trick

Using a variation of the Wait for the Hangover Trick will enhance your success—gives you a way to change up if needed. Say you've held your peace for a while, held back your helpful suggestions, waiting for a time when you are almost sure to get through to him. While he is mentally handicapped, hung-over, arrange yourself to look him in the face.

1. Say something like this: "I know you don't feel well, __(use his name here)__ but I need to tell you something. I have a problem with _____ (fill in the blank). Make it something he did *this* time—*never from a previous time* because it allows him to shut you out. He'll slam down to voice his protest.

2. Now Breathe. A brief pause creates a space for what you said to sink in.

3. Count to three before adding, "What can you do about this?"

> **Psych Note:** When you ask him to do something from now on, use "Will you" rather than "Can you." "Will you" goes into his subconscious differently than "Can you."
> "Will you" lights up a different kind of attention. He cannot

> rebel against this as well as "Can you," because "Can you" carries an underlying test of his manhood, his ability.
> "   Will you" distracts him from his self-centered misery, calls on his manhood and anything good that's still there.)

4. **No Smile,** Move Along. Smoothly leave the area Immediately. Disappear. Do not respond to any questions or comments. If you leave it as is, it will, will! get through. If you can leave the house, do so. Often, feeling alone and abandoned sets the stage for him to think about what just happened.

5. In any case, immediately go do something fun—away from his area. Give yourself a break—even if short. Do or think only what is pleasant, dumping thoughts about him and his behavior for the moment. This is time for you to get back your balance. While, I might add, he and his subconscious mull over his predicament! If possible, stay scarce for at least 30 minutes.

(Note: Before you use the Wait for the Hangover Trick, write the words you want to you say when you get the opportunity. Go back over them at least three times to
improve on improve the way you describe the problem;
improve how you tell him what change you want to see;
improve the way your voice sounds and what you want to emphasize;
improve your posture to look composed and self-confident.
If you practice these things now, you'll be ready and do great when the time comes.)

* * *

MASTERY

Pull out one or two points from this chapter that you especially want to absorb fast and write them here.

1. _____

_____

2. _____

_____

Chapter 5

Where you
  find out whether he has a real problem
  find out how far it has progressed
  *find **much** food for thought*

Wanna Know How Bad His Drinking Problem Really Is?

Ever wonder if he's "a real alcoholic"? Wanna know for sure?

If he has a problem, would you like to know just how bad it really is?

This is the chapter gives you your answers. And the checklist in this chapter is sufficient to convince everyone else too—even him—of what's really going on. Let's get to it!

Your checklist gives more value if you understand the basics of the disorder you've been dealing with. You've come a long way in that to arrive at this page of the book. You can build your understanding still more and be enriched by it, starting here:

We can already say with confidence that he definitely has a disorder. We can say that because it's disrupting his life and he doesn't change! And he's disrupting your life, someone he claims to love, but he doesn't change. Worse: He cannot stop drinking the elixir that is slowly eating away his brain.

Since it attacks first the part of his brain that can see and assess this, he is helpless at times, sick at times, dense and stupid at times.

You've absorbed by now that his worsening behavior and your worsening relationship problems are both directly connected to his drinking. But you're still not sure how bad his problem really is.

Let's talk a bit about the upcoming checklist. This checklist tells you what stage he's in, and that's valuable information because it points to the best approach, as well as the best treatment.

Another value of the following list of signs of drinking problems is that you'll get a better idea of what to do about your situation when you get a better idea of how bad his problem is—what stage he's in, and his chances of actually recovering.

If he's in the Early Stage, there's some hope, but in the more progressed stages, your chances of effective help to get him to change are nil. That's the Bad News. On the other hand, it's also Very Good News to you.

"*What?*" you may be thinking.

Yep. Knowing he's beyond the stage where he's most likely to change really is Good News. Here's why: Once you really, truly, confidently know that trying to "fix" him is less than useless (less than useless because it's actually harmful—to you) you will be able to stop all obsessing. Once you know he's extremely unlikely to accept help and stay with it, you don't need to obsess anymore about what to do and how to do it. With a solid assessment of his true condition, you don't have to be frustrated with him ever again. And that's because you get frustrated when you try to do something that keeps being blocked. Knowing that he's beyond the point where your efforts will do much good sets you free. You know in advance y our attempts won't work.

You'll also shed your own special denial (the kind you share with 20 or 30 million other women in the United States alone, with countless millions of others around the world). You and they practice a form of partial denial, which boils down to being unable to accept he is as hopeless as your observations tell you. A part of you knows he's beyond fixing, but a bigger part still believes that if you love him enough (Belle and the Beast) you will awaken him from his condition (a reverse Snow White).

You'll recall that psychological "denial" is mentally shutting out something that threatens to overwhelm you. Denial isn't a bad thing. Wired in by the Manufacturer as a survival tool, denial is a reflex action your brain takes to protect you (itself) when events become too big to cope with. Don't think you've been bad or you're mentally disordered for being in denial of how truly bad your situation ma be.

(Note: I've decided that denial is also part of what I call Bambi-Brain, another form of full or partial brain freeze.)

Your subconscious, amidst its billions of other processes, also keeps tabs on your minute-by-minute levels of strength and balance, so it knows what you are capable of handling at any given moment. It's possible to overrule its decisions by firmly ignoring its signals, and that is what you have been doing much of the time with his problem. And you've done it solely because of the caring, strong, giving, loving person you are (most of the time—until you're pushed too far).

Denial gives you the ability to shut off or minimize your awareness of threatening events; it saves you from being overwhelmed and made helpless, Bambi-Brained, where you can't function at all to protect yourself. Being overwhelmed creates helplessness, so your wired-in denial system lets you focus on small portions of a problem at a time, and it falls out of your focus completely at times. And you survive. But you're not happy. Denial, minimizing or dodging a problem, has a bad name currently, but its intended purpose is quite important. When it overrides a reality that can become life- or mind-threatening, it's bad. When it allows you to escape mental anguish briefly, it is good—say, times when a loved one has died.

You can see that Denial is basically a protective brain function "Denial" parcels out your ability to take in a full situation to avoid overwhelming you and making you totally helpless..

If you didn't have this Manufacturer-installed denial system, you'd live in a constant state of Bambi Brain because life is full of potential harm. (And, of course, potential good, but that's not pertinent at the moment.)

Most of you have never wanted to believe your guy was becoming a wreck, unsalvageable. At this point in this book, you know that it's possible. He may be a wreck, heading ever faster into absolute self-destruction, running right over everything close in the process. And you are learning that it's possible that he has little hope of pulling out of it. Some, but very little.

Maybe you still love him, or maybe your position is such that he is an important element of your own best interests. Denial is more comfortable when you contemplate how you can cope with the consequences of his disorder. You may more easily recognize denial working in you if you recall times you've gotten just so far into looking for a solution, and then thrown up your hands and stolen Scarlet O'Hara's line: Well, I'll worry about that tomorrow.

It can feel like a phantom gust of wind. Poof. Your mind jumps to coping with something else. To keep it at bay a part of you has to begin shutting out events, flashing on them then jumping away because "they are just too much to deal with right now. I'll get back to this later."

You intelligently know, consciously, that just because you don't *want* to know something doesn't make it go away. But denial is subconscious, so it can play with magic. Without conscious interference, it is capable of running the whole show—getting you focused on things outside the immediate catastrophe. The coming checklist is going to get you back in reality, provide you a conscious intervention.

> **Psych Note:** "Denial" is a full or partial closing of the mind to thought about a threatening reality.

Most women resist labeling their mate as "alcoholic," even when they've read the signs and recognized that he has them. This is denial at work.

Knowing the stage of a drinker's problem makes it possible to give him the form of treatment with the best chance of working. This approach, however, doesn't exist in any current treatment approach I've investigated to date.

The questionnaire you'll be using includes some items similar to those on other lists, but it goes far beyond earlier models. Professionals currently are forced to use the existing, inadequate, guidelines. We cannot receive insurance payment for services unless the "patient" is diagnosed along these inadequate, ineffective lines. In fact, a professional can lose her licenses for not using these inadequate, ineffective guidelines. Extending the diagnostic criteria to allow for earlier intervention is the entire reason I created this list of items in the first place.

Brain scans find holes in the brains of over-drinkers; how big they are varies mostly with how long they have been drinking. This fact is not included as a primary diagnostic. It's not a huge intellectual leap to start looking for such signs that show themselves long before those holes in the brain get so huge the sufferer hasn't the brain power left to escape his dreadful consequence.

Not surprisingly, a number of mental health practitioners tell me they are on board with expanding the list of signs that mark the deterioration of an over-drinker. Their reason: Using it will allow needed treatment far earlier in the destruction of his life. And brain.

Although no fixed "line" marks where a drinker changes from nice guy to horse's butt, we can allowing earlier diagnosis by an expanded tracking of deterioration serious drinkers have in common, thus saving lives—of drinkers and their partners.

Most people continue to hold the idea that until one is jobless, homeless, sick, weak, and disreputable he isn't "alcoholic," although the alcohol problem is off to a flying start in all people with their very first drink! And that is not due to the drinker's weak will; it's due to the action of alcohol on body and brain cells. For those with a genetic setup for it, this brain cell destruction accrues faster.

While the potential for "alcoholism" commences at the very first drink, a number of events marking movement in that direction can be used as markers. These markers signal that a drinker is caught in the trap and sinking, the trap that allows escape to fewer than 10 percent of those who fall into it.

While alcohol deadens, then kills, nerve cells (especially brain cells), that's not the worst of it. The worst of it is that the first and hardest hit brain cells happen to be in critical portions of the brain: the brain areas responsible for judgement, including judging whether he's had enough to drink! The decision-making area is affected accordingly, warping judgements like whether to put on the brakes now, or whether to shut up now, or refuse a drink. Bad judgement sounds like: "I'm not too drunk to drive.

Then there are the brain cells making up his memory: Short-term memory is located in one of the areas first hit by alcohol. Once he takes a drink, he forgets that he just decided he was going to quit. Perhaps more importantly, he forgets his reasons for not wanting to drink too much.

He forgets how many he's had so he's unsure when he reaches the limit he's set. He forgets how much his family means to him. He forgets his marriage vows.

As the alcohol load in his blood picks up, being disposed of far slower than it's being refilled, all brain cells slug down. First injured, numbed and slowed, then wounded, then dying—and no treatment known today restores a damaged or dead brain cell.

The information each injured and dying brain cell holds evaporates. Even if brain cells did grow back, the replacements wouldn't hold the information encoded in the originals. Just growing new cells wouldn't give him access to earlier memories.

Memory: A promise to be home in time for dinner; remembering how bad a hangover feels; all of his vows never to do it again.

The coming checklist has hundreds of signs—so many that it is impossible for a diagnostician to miss a developing drinking problem. Research has already shown that all of the signs listed accompany a progressing drinking problem. I wonder if there were so many signs of heart trouble, would a diagnostic guide leave off hundreds of other signs that could save the life?

I've made sure the signs I've listed are observable; that means anyone could see them. (Of course, no one sees all of the action behind the scenes except those who live with him. While anyone could see them, most are vigorously hidden by the drinker and rarely seen—until the bitter end—except by the drinker's mate. (Even she won't see it all, as most of you already know. Over-drinkers are masters at hiding what they do.)

While some of the "pre-drink" signs may not be directly observable by the drinker's woman, she usually knows about, for instance, other heavy drinkers in the family line and many of his early drinking escapades. (Again I point out: Doctors ask about heart problems and cancer in the family and use those to make their diagnoses of this person. Not about drinking though.)

(Note: As to heredity, the drinking problem sometimes "skips" generations, only to pop up again later. Like blue eyes or red hair. Someone once said that if "alcoholism" isn't hereditary, it must be contagious! That's because so many in families develop the problem.

Signs you'll see listed here include those seen in the very Early Stage. Usually, these signs are dismissed as "just part of drinking," or "just a young man sowing his oats." The sure warning these signs show goes unheeded. (If these problems are "just part of growing up," how do you explain the billions of young men who grow up without creating such experiences?)

For those who continue to drink more than the one to three drinks per 24 hours—over-drinking—only trouble lies ahead. Yet it can be headed off years before the drinker has destroyed everything around him. That's why we must begin spotting it earlier. It's like catching a transmittable disease before it has a chance to destroy.

We have learned in all other health disorders, the sooner spotted, the more likely prevented and remedied. No physician finding a lump in your breast, no matter how small, fears he shouldn't diagnose sufficiently to allow for further testing. The physician doesn't decide that diagnosis should wait until the lump is a certain size, or crosses some "line" before taking it seriously.

Whether lumps, vascular irregularities, or signs of infection, physicians immediately set up further exams and discuss early intervention with the patient.

But not with over-drinking.

Most professionals can't know about (they're not published, taught, or given prescriptive therapy for) using the early signs of a problem destined for hell to help the patient. To do this, the partner's input, assessment, is far more reliable than anything the patient will say. Listen to him—but rather than buying in, concentrate on ways you can help him see his reality.

Making it harder for a physician or counselor to see the reality of an over-drinker is that even in an early stage, he's rarely going to tell the truth about how much he drinks for fear of being cut off from it.

Professionals must start relying on outside observations, interview the people close to the drinker in order to make a valid diagnosis. It's similar to the way we work with children. We get input about their behaviors from their parents, their teachers, other counselors who have been involved with him. This is the approach required to help the over-drinker.

> *The least reliable person in the world to accurately report the truth about his drinking is the drinker.*
>
> *The most reliable person for information about his drinking, especially the worst of it, is his mate. (But even she doesn't know all of it, the worst of it, because he hides it from her, and he'll likely try to hide it from the professional.)*

A physician is not concerned that a lump could turn out to be a false sign so she doesn't say anything or advise treatment! To the contrary, the physician hopes it will turn out to be nothing. (And the insurance company does too.)

Yet none of the disorders currently better treated causes the disruption and destruction of the lives of everyone the patient touches like over-drinking. Most professionals continue to hold back saying what needs to be said out of fear of error, or losing a patient—as well as having the cultural vague sense of having no right to pry into someone's drinking. Professionals! Get over it!

Numerous books have been written about and for caretakers of chronically ill persons—all with a strong focus on how the stress of their relationship with the impaired person affects them. But no such book has been written for the partners of an over-drinker. Until now. Here it is, my darlings.

I hope that this chapter and its questionnaire give you the information you need for your future interactions with him. You, the drinker's woman, are likely the only person on earth who sees those early signs—(and a great many of those that follow). You may already have experienced resistance getting friends and family (his family mostly) to see that he has a problem. Sometimes his family and friends point to you as the problem. I mean, what else could they think: It's what he tells them (and they do see you—stressed, angry, maybe edgy. Even when his problem and its consequent behaviors become blatant, many remain in denial. "It's really not that bad." (Meaning: "The lump doesn't yet weight a full pound so ignore it!")

All questions on the coming checklist address signs of over-drinking that anyone very close to the drinker can see. The drinker, however, allows fewer and fewer people that close. On their own, a sign may mean little, but when they appear together, there's a problem—current or in the making. I listed the many signs roughly in the order they *usually* occur. While not all drinkers do all the listed things, or in precisely in the same order, all over-drinkers will do most of these things in roughly the same order. That's because alcohol damages brain cells the same way in most people. Brain cells change or die in the same brain areas, producing nearly the same behaviors in over-drinkers. Like tuberculosis, where the same kind of damage occurs in the same organ of people who have it, with about the same result. Death, if not treated adequately.

Some drinkers can skip chunks of signs on this list, jumping from Early Middle Stage signs straight into End Stage signs, hence, when you come to a string of items that seem not to apply, don't stop there. Continue assessing items to the very end. Some drinkers anchor at a level, maybe for years, before observable changes start appearing again.

There is a second reason for continuing on down the list of signs. Because brain damage causes behavioral change the same in all over-drinkers, looking at signs further along shows you what to expect. Knowing what's coming also tunes your subconscious to pick up on them when they begin occurring. You won't miss them.

It is possible for an over-drinker to leap over some markers of downfall and rush far ahead into more advanced levels.

This most often occurs when something especially bad happens to him—getting a terminal disease, death of a loved one, loss of a job or career, financial ruin, or other such tragedies. He's already drinking (and already has a problem in the cooker), but because alcohol brings mental and emotional relief (temporarily), he will turn to it, and step it up. This is why many people think it was the bad event that caused his problem—but he already had the problem before the bad event. The bad event simply speeded up his deterioration.

An over-drinker "knows" how to relieve his mental discomfort-and emotional pain. Drinkers who have held the line for a long time will seek that relief more often after an unhappiness. His drinking picks up, his deterioration takes him down.

I've heard many drinkers's women say that they feel guilty for not really caring a lot if he gets injured or commits suicide. In fact, many admit to flashes of maybe being relieved should it happen. Who can blame them? I ask you: Is it bad to wish the guy firing cannon balls at you would drop dead? No, of course not. Those feelings are actually normal! They prove you are normal. Drop any guilty feelings.

Attention! Remember--An over-drinker drinks for only one reason: the feeling it gives him. He doesn't drink because he had a hard day, or because you were mean to him. He drinks because when things happen that he doesn't like and make him feel bad, he has discovered a way to change that—fast. His subconscious took over from there. It works the same with chocolate cake, smoking, drugs, gambling, sexual adventures (sounds fun when I say it like that!), with prescription and other drugs.

His dependence on this way of getting relief, coupled with specific cells of his body actually becoming dependent on a goodly supply of alcohol add up to addiction in its fullest form.

Body cells must adjust to large amounts of alcohol when drinking picks up; they must change their makeup to cope. When the alcohol stops, they are in distress because they have changed to function with it. Without it, they don't work well. This, combined with the actual poisoning of his body with over-drinking are what's going on when he has a hangover.

When his intake of alcohol stops, every cell in his body begins will cry out for it. Having altered themselves over time, these cells growing a little here, shrinking a little there, producing less of whatever the cell produces because the alcohol begins takes its place in the . The cell has adjusted to accommodate loads of alcohol, and like a balloon that has been stretched too far now hangs slack and useless because they now need alcohol to function.

These body cells set up an inner scream like nothing else can—except much the same cells for hard drugs

* * *

Ready, Set? . . .

Go to the bathroom, then get coffee or tea, or whatever works for you, find a quiet space where you can work for the next hour or so without interruption. (It's not the end of the world if you get interrupted; it just means you have to hunker down later to regain your level of concentration.)

Now, pencil in hand, read each item, each one a sign commonly seen in problem drinkers. Not all signs will appear in all drinkers, and not all will appear in exactly the same order. If you have observed a sign in your drinker (or know it is fact) put a checkmark by it.

The checklist is for you—not a judge, not the evening news. You can share it later if you wish, especially with his physician, but its purpose is just for you to get an idea of what's going on with him, for you to diagnose (roughly) how far the problem that is ripping your life apart has progressed.

Relax as you answer the questions. You aren't swearing to your answers in a court of law!

Now will missing a few, or checking a few incorrectly won't make a big difference in your final outcome.

STAGE ONE

THE PRE-DRINKING STAGE
(His Genetic and Physical set-up)

___1. Did (do) either of his parents drink too much?
___2. Did (do) any of his siblings drink too much?
___3. Did (do) any of his grandparents drink too much?
___4. Did (do) any of his great-grandparents drink too much?
___5. Did (do) any of his blood-related aunts or uncles drink too much?
___6. Is he over 40 years old?
___7. Is he under 24 years old? (Age 24 is approximately when the brain stops growing. Until then, it's is still growing, thus susceptible to far more damage than it will a few years later.)

* * *

STAGE TWO

THE EARLY STAGES
(Even if your guy is beyond the early stages and no longer does these things, if he did them in the past, check them.)

Early Early Stage

___8. Is there a change in his personality when drinking?
___9. Does (or did) he seem to "hold his liquor" better than others do in the early days?
___10. Does he drink fast?

____11. Does he appear to look forward to drinking events?
____12. Does he talk about drinking as if it's a lot of fun?
____13. Does he enjoy leisure activities less where he can't include drinking?

(A thought to contemplate: If you've seen him drink an entire six-pack, think: Does he ever sit down and drink a six-pack of spring water? Or cola?)

____14. Does he act grandiose when drinking?
____15. When he drinks, does he drink more than the U.S. National Institutes of Health says is the safe amount?
____16. Does he drink more than others with him?
____17. When most others quit, does he continue?
____18. Does (did) his sex drive increase when drinking early on?
____19. Has anyone ever said "He seems to have a hollow leg"?
____20. Does he drink until he gets drunk?
____21. Is he moody, depressed, easily angered, jumpy, or sick after drinking the night before?
____22. Does he go on to drink again after suffering for it (either a bad hangover or some other negative experience that was connected to his drinking)?
____23. Has he ever appeared not to remember any part of his drinking time?

Mid-Early Stage

(Be sure to take note of the first item of each stage; that item is the sign moving him up from one level to the next.)

____24. Did he go back and drink again, continue to drink (and over-drink) after experiencing bad events associated with his drinking?
____25. Do certain events (or feelings) seem to trigger him to think about getting a drink?
____26. Does he use excuses to drink (and over-drink) like "I had a bad day," or "It's the President's birthday" ?
____27. Has he become more critical of others?
____28. Does he seem to look forward to getting a drink, as if it is a party or a reward? (Like at the end of a work day or his work week.)
____29. Does he seem to look forward to social gatherings where

there will be drinking?
____30. Does he appear uncomfortable if he cannot drink at social gatherings?
____31. Has his behavior when drinking ever embarrassed you?
____32. Does (or did) he do foolish or dangerous things when drinking?
____33. When fixing drinks, does he sneak an extra pop, or a whole drink?
____34. Is he more boisterous when drinking?
____35. Does he drink more in amount now than in the past?
____36. Does he drink more often now than in the past?
____37. Does he buy more alcohol now than in the past?
____38. Does he neglect food, or eat less, when drinking?
____39. Have you complained about things that he does while he's drinking?

Late Early Stage
(Again—note the first item, the signal he's moved deeper.)

____40. Did the behaviors you complained about continue to be a problem?
____41. Or did they stop for a while, but then come back?
____42. Have you complained to him about how much he drinks, or how often?
____43. After you complained, did he try to cut down or quit?
____44. Did he get irritable because you complained?
____45. Did he continue to drink anyway or, if he decided to cut down or quit, did he eventually go back to it?
____46. Has he ever excused something he did by saying, "I only did that because I was drunk"? (This item shows that he loses control when drinking, otherwise he wouldn't do something drinking that he would not do otherwise.)
____47. Has he ever changed his routine to have more opportunities for drinking? (Like getting together with friends or joining a new group of friends.)
____48. Does he act uncomfortable (or disturbed) when you talk to him about his drinking?
____49. Has he said he wanted a drink to relax, unwind, chill, loosen up, forget the bad day or event? (Drinking to get a specific feeling. Saying it shows he knows it's unusual.)
____50. Has he said any of those things more than once?

____51. Is he having money problems, yet he continues to spend money on drinking?
____52. Does he drink to calm down when upset?
____53. When talking about drinking, does he say "I'm going to have a drink," when he'll surely have more than one?
____54. Has he ever planned or promised to drink only a certain amount, then went ahead and had more than that amount? (This is a sign of loss of control.)
____55. Has he ever planned not to drink at all at some event, then did anyway?
____56. Has he ever failed to keep a commitment due to something associated with his drinking?
____57. Has he said he doesn't want to drink before a specific time of day?
____58. Has he tried to cut down on his drinking on his own?
____59. Did his attempt to cut down eventually fail?
____60. Has he said he felt badly about his drinking, or things he had done when drinking?

* * *

STAGE THREE - MIDDLE STAGES
Early Middle Stage
(Again, note the item marking his step-up
to a more serious stage.)

____61. Having said that he feels bad about his behavior when he was drinking, did he then go on to drink again?
____62. Has he ever been drinking (or over-drinking) at an inappropriate time?
____63. Has he become more critical of others (including you), even when not drinking?
____64. Does he often dodge his responsibility for when bad things happen (especially those occurring when he was drinking)? (Usually this happens by his blaming others.)
____65. Is he evasive about how much, how often, with whom, where, or other information about his drinking?
____66. Is drinking interfering with his hobbies or sports so that he's doing less of things he used to enjoy?
____67. Has he made you give excuses to anyone for his

behavior, or his absences, due to over-drinking?
____68. Has he made a rule to do most of his drinking at home?
____69. Did he eventually break his own rule?
____70. Has he promised to drink less at home, but eventually started drinking as much again?
____71. When you confronted him about drinking more, did he start drinking more often away from home? (Where his behavior couldn't be tracked as well by your lying eyes?)
____72. Has he become upset when prevented from going to a drinking event?
____73. Does he avoid family members who don't drink?
____74. Does he avoid friends who don't drink?
____75. Does he select mostly entertainment that allows drinking?
____76. As a couple, do you not associate with friends as much anymore because of his drinking, or his behavior?
____77. Has he lied to anyone about his drinking?
____78. Has he begun staying out later drinking?
____79. Has he changed the type of drinks he drinks (such as from liquor to beer, or beer to light beer) in an attempt to cut down his drinking?
____80. Does he get defensive or argumentative if someone other than you talks to him about his drinking?
____81. Do friends say that they think he's drinking too much?
____82. Has his spending associated with drinking (or drinking behavior) begun to drain the family?
____83. Has he become more self-centered?
____84. Does he speak of wanting to "get drunk"?
____85. Have you ever spoken to a family member about your concerns over his drinking?
____86. Does he drink when angry?
____87. Does he often seem unable to remember everything that happened while he was drinking?
____88. Has he ever asked someone what happened during any of the time he was drinking?
____89. Has he, when drinking, ever hurt your feelings (or other people's)?
____90. Has he promised not to do it again, but then has done it again when drinking?
____91. Has he ever tried to quit drinking?

Mid-Middle Stage
(Note the first item. It signals another step down.)

____91. Did his attempt to quit drinking fail?
____92. Has he begun to lose interest in things he used to enjoy?
____93. Has he become more aggressive when drinking or hungover?
____94. Has his behavior embarrassed you?
____95. Has he started arguments with you while drinking?
____96. Has he started arguments with others when drinking?
____97. Have you talked to one of your friends about his drinking?
____98. Does he drink when others do not?
____99. Is his drinking causing other problems in the home?
____100. Has he neglected an obligation—work, family, health, job, or appointments—due to drinking or something associated with his drinking?
____101. Has he missed an important appointment or event due to drinking or something associated with drinking?
____102. Has he hidden or lied to you about his drinking, especially concerning the amount?
____103. Does he become more restless when he's not drinking?
____104. Has he said that a drink helps him get away from pressures for a while? (Changing his feelings.)
____105. Has he ever mentioned wondering if he had a drinking problem?
____106. Does he spend a lot of time drinking?
____107. Has he ever set a limit on how much to drink at home or an event, or any other time?
____108. Has he gone beyond a limit he set? (Sign of inability to control his drinking.)
____109. Does he hurt you emotionally or become verbally abusive when he is drinking?
____110. Has he left an argument with you to get a drink or go out drinking?
____111. Has he ever been in trouble with his job or work due to something associated with drinking?
____112. Does he plan things but not follow through (more than in the past)?
____113. Does he start on projects, then drop them (more than in the past)?

____114. Are you unsure about how much he's drinking now?
____115. Has he taken up a hobby/sport to help him cut down on his drinking?
____115. Did that attempt eventually fail?
____116. Has he changed his usual drink to boost the kick? Or use drugs, legal or illegal, to do that?
____117. Has he changed his type of alcoholic drink to help him cut down and control his drinking?
____118. Has that tactic failed to help him cut down (and stay cut down)? (The beginning of loss of control.)
____119. Does he get into arguments with others in social settings, such as at parties?
____120. Has he lost friends due to his drinking?
____121. Has he kept a "stash" of alcohol in a place where he could get a drink secretly?
____122. Have family members asked you to get him to cut down or to quit?
____123. Has he ever seen a list of signs of a drinking problem and been argumentative or sarcastic about them?
____124. Has he recognized that he has signs of a problem, but continued drinking?
____125. Does he drink when bored?
____126. Has he changed his routine to help him cut down his drinking?
____127. Have his changes eventually failed to work?
____128. Has he made more than one serious attempt to quit?
____129. Did these attempts fail?
____130. Has he left a specific group of people in an attempt to cut down on his drinking?
____131. Did it fail to keep him cut down-quit?
____132. Have you ever found liquor he'd watered down to make the bottle appear fuller, or a totally replaced a bottle for the same reason?
____133. Has he been in physical fights when drinking?
____134. When he controls his drinking for some special occasion, does he soon afterward drink more?
____135. Has there been more than one time he confessed to bad behavior, or expressed remorse for his behavior while drinking?
____136. Was his expression of guilt or remorse completely believable?
____137. Did he go back to drink again?

____138. Has he ever left a job in order to cut down or quit drinking?
____139. Did that change eventually fail?
____140. Has he ever moved to another neighborhood or town in an attempt to get a new start, to cut down or quit drinking?
____141. Did that attempt eventually fail?
____142. Have you suspected that your drinker sets up arguments just to get an excuse to go drinking?

Late Middle Stage

____143. Does he drink when he's alone?
____144. Does he take one or two drinks fast, to get started?
____145. Has he ever been arrested for anything associated with drinking?
____146. Has he continued to drink after the arrest?
____147. Has he suffered illness because of drinking?
____148. Has he continued to drink even so?
____149. Do you believe he is dependent on alcohol?
____150. Has his physical health continued to deteriorate?
____151. Have you suspected he was lying when he claimed no memory of something done while drinking?
____152. Does he seem to have less fun when drinking now than in the past?
____153. Has his personality changed even when he's not drinking?
____154. Do you see physical signs of heavy drinking—broken veins, bloodshot eyes, looking tired or older, a swollen upper belly, slackened muscles?
____155. Has he ever gone off a medication, or decided not to take a medication, because he could not drink alcohol while taking it?
____156. Does he have decreased sex drive (or ability)?
____157. Does he seem bored (or restless) more than in the past?
____158. Has he—who never harmed or threatened you or your children before--when drinking threatened or committed such harm?
____159. Has he threatened you more than once?
____160. Has he threatened to harm you when he was not drinking?
____161. Has he ever hurt you physically, or been violent with you?

If you answered "yes" to the last question, it is extremely important for you to seek qualified professional help as soon as possible, and certainly before trying to discuss any of this with him: A women's hotline counselor is your best bet, but a licensed mental health counselor, licensed social worker, or your health professional all can give you information to help keep you safe or set you up with others who can. If he has ever been violent, get direction from the professionals before talking to him about what you find. Also, keep in mind that there's really no need to talk to him about it. This man may be far beyond fixing with a talk.

You absolutely are not safe if you live with a problem drinker who ever becomes in the least violent. His behavior control is steadily slipping. This means you cannot predict when it will fail completely.

Staying free of crippling injuries, or losing your life—whether he meant to do it or not—depends on being aware, staying observant, and getting a qualified professional to guide you from here.

____162. Is his over-all physical condition continuing to deteriorate?

____163. Does he spend more time alone?

____164. Has he started drinking with people considered of a lower class than him?

____165. Does he flirt with other women while drinking?

____166. Have his morals slipped in other ways?

____167. Does he frequently talk about or show an excess of worry or fear?

____168. Has he begun having vision problems—especially night vision? (Alcohol can affect vision.)

____169. Does he seem to have long periods during drinking that he can't remember?

____170. Have other family members shown concern about his drinking?

____171. Does he blame others for his problems or for his over-drinking?

____172. Has he become almost continually critical of others?

____173. Has he ever made a show of leaving a little of his drink unfinished? (What normal drinker would do that?)

____174. Has he continued drinking all night?

____175. Has he begun to suffer high levels of anxiety or panic attacks, or spells of deep depression?
____176. Does he ever drink early in his day--before noon (or the equivalent if on shift work)?
____177. Does he drink the morning after over-drinking?
____178. Does he take a drink to ease a hangover?
____179. Has he become more jealous?
____180. Do you suspect him of sexual misbehavior?
____181. Have you suspected (or known) that your drinker has been sexually unfaithful?
____182. Does he appear to have memory problems even when not drinking?
____183. Has he ever drunk while on the job?
____184. Has he threatened to find somebody else (another woman) who understands him?
____185. Has he ever lost a job because of anything associated with his drinking?
____186. Has his job or other important source of his welfare suggested that he go for counseling?
____187. Has he gone for any type of counseling—or mental health treatment?
____188. Did he drop or discontinue treatment?
____188. Has he told you (or do you suspect) that when he saw a counselor or doctor, he was not honest about his drinking?
____189. Has he begun taking medication for anxiety, or sleep medications? (Anxiety and sleep disorder accompany a growing drinking problem.)
____190. Has anyone ever called the police on him when he was drinking—even if he was innocent of the charge.
____191. Has he continued drinking despite that?
____192. Has he stopped or lessened expressing remorse for bad behavior?
____193. Does he become verbally abusive (or shut you out completely) when you talk about his drinking?
____194. Has he ever been injured seriously enough to require medical care associated with his drinking?
____195. Has he been hospitalized due to drinking or something associated with his drinking?
____196. Did he return to drinking after that?
____197. Does he seem antsy when wanting to get a drink?
____198. Is he having flashes of intense emotion—especially anger, fear, or jealousy—whether drinking or not?

____199. Has he had an automobile accident when drinking or hung-over?
____200. Has he ever been the driver, while drinking or hung-over, when someone else was injured?
____201. After that accident, did he resume drinking at the same rate as before?
____203. Has he ever been arrested, or taken to jail for something associated with drinking?
____204. After getting out of jail, did he resume drinking?
____205. Have you seen signs of further diminishing health—he's paler, thinning hair, sexual problems, wasting away or packing on fat, broken veins on his face, easy bruising?
____206. Does he react with anger to your pointing out his health effects (perhaps going for a drink afterward)?
____207. Has he argued or become hostile when anyone else has tried to talk to him about his drinking, behavior, or health?
_☐_208. Have you begun to seek help for either him or yourself? (I checked this one for you. You're doing that by reading this book.)
____209. Have you spoken to a counselor or doctor about your partner's drinking?
____210. Has he ever been charged with drunk driving?
____211. After that charge, did he eventually resume drinking?
____212. Has he ever been open, even briefly, to getting any kind of help for the drinking?
____213. Does he seem to have frequent bouts of remorse?
____214. Does he have more than one hidden alcohol stash?
____215. Has he occasionally shown signs of wanting to get back into church, or other signs of spiritual hunger?
____216. Has your partner ever gone to a counselor, physician, or minister specifically for help with his drinking?
____217. Has he ever been in jail overnight or longer for something associated with drinking (different from just going to jail and bonding out)?
____218. Did he continue drinking after that?
____219. Has he ever attended a meeting of Alcoholics Anonymous?
____220. Does he ever say he hates himself?
____221. Have his testicles or penis shrunk? (BTW--Over-drinking causes male genitals to shrink, often first seen in his testicles.)

* * *

STAGE FOUR

END STAGE

____222. Has he ever been hospitalized for mental health or substance abuse treatment?
____223. After treatment, did he eventually start drinking?
____224. He's used up his excuses for over-drinking; he no longer gives excuses when he drinks.
____225. Have almost all family and friends backed away from him?
____226. Does he continue to drink, despite illnesses or health warnings?
____227. Has he sought out spiritual help, but it failed to stop the drinking (for good)?
____228. Has he stopped making plans to do anything?
____229. Do his hands shake, especially early in his day?
____230. Do you notice tremors in his hands, voice, even his knees, when he's not drinking?
____231. Have you noticed that shakes diminish or disappear for a while after he takes a drink?
____232. Does he ever appear unsteady when walking, even when not drinking?
____233. Does he spend most of his time (off work) isolated and drinking (at home or in a favorite bar)?
____234. Has he committed a felony when drinking?
____235. Has he served a jail/prison sentence?
____236. Has he continued drinking after that?
____237. Does he have any type of liver trouble?
____238. Does he have any pancreas trouble?
____239. Has he ever vomited blood (dark red or bright red)?
____240. Does he continue to drink despite serious health issues?
____241. Does he have difficulty sleeping—unable to asleep for more than a few hours at a time?

____242. Does he get up and drink to get back to sleep?
____243. Does he have a swollen, hard upper belly?
____244. Is he drinking less alcohol at a sitting now, but he still seems to get drunk?
____245. Does he have an illness that can kill him if he continues drinking?
____246. Does he continue to drink even so?
____247. Has he made more than one attempt at getting help?
____248. Did he return to drinking?
____249. Has he said he-others would be better off if he were dead?
____250. Has he ever threatened suicide?
____251. Has he been hospitalized for any illness associated with or aggravated by his drinking?
____252. Did he start drinking again after that?
____253. Does he seem to have given up on changing?
____254. Has he ever said he doesn't care if something kills him—like an accident, his health, the drinking?
____255. Has he ever said he hopes something kills him?
____256. Has he attempted to kill himself?
____257. Has he attempted to kill someone else—even if he says he wasn't serious (or was "just drunk")?
____258. Has he become vegetative, sitting or sleeping much of the time if not working?
____259. Is he frequently incoherent or impossible to talk to because he's drunk?
____261. Did he actually commit suicide? Or has he died of other causes associated with his drinking?

Okay. That's it!
You've done well. Good Girl!
(Pat yourself on the butt, smile and say, "Good Girl!" to yourself.)

You now have a lot of factual material to work with, more I trust than you did when you picked up this book.
No matter what you discover on this checklist, you are bound to have millions (many millions!) of sisters in the United States alone whose drinkers are in more or less the same stages. That

means they will be going through more or less the same things you are dealing with. Again--you are not alone! I guarantee you that all of you can be of great help to one another, which is the reason for our blog.

This is a great time to take a short break—even overnight, let all this information begin to settle in. Or—you can keep right on! It's your decision.

* * *

What Is This Chapter's Check-List Telling You?

Having this questionnaire to work with means that you don't need a professional to diagnose him and know what's going on. You may, however, need a professional or a trained women's hotline counselor to help you decide what's best and safest for you to do about it, given your current circumstances.

The behaviors that you just examined are all signs that would be observable to anyone—especially anyone as close to the drinker as you are. (As you've likely also observed, over-drinkers are very clever at hiding their true condition from others.)

Based on your checkmarks:

Do you think he has a drinking problem? _____

If so, what stage is indicated? _____

What does the checklist suggest likely comes next on his way down?

1. _____

2. _____

3. _____

* * *

You have absorbed a load of information, mostly information I know you were looking for. Others before you have used what they have learned up to this point to understand their drinker's situation, and to understand their own position. Most have used this information to make decisions about what to do **based on what's best for them—not the drinker.**

Many of your rare and beautiful sisters have based their life decisions at this point back on the dream or wish that the drinker will get better. Also on the belief they really can change another person *and make them stay changed.*

I hope that every one of you who want to remain in your relationship or in your home will be able to do so. The information and tricks here will be a big help. The information you've gained this far puts you in a much better position to consider your future paths, to consider and weigh out your own best interests, to make the best decision you can at that moment (which is truly the best anyone can ever do).

Making any decision or change at this point will likely be difficult, likely painful. And you may find out as you try to follow through that you're not able to—at least not immediately. Not doing anything is also painful; I would say not doing anything can be more painful. Making a decision doesn't cure the problem; it only gives you a focus that will like take you closer to your cure, step by step..

If you can help the drinker without sacrificing yourself, by all means do so. Be watchful *not* to sacrifice your own best interests in the hope your sacrifice will work. It won't. Look at the record. Backing up a step here leaves you less to bargain with later too.

Both your conscious and subconscious mind(s) will continue processing all the things you have taken in. Bit by bit it will fall in place to soon seem natural and normal. This means you can relax now and let things fall into place as they do; let up any push—unless your situation is dangerous. Don't try to force anything if you don't have to for safety's sake.

Get busy, get active—do something, preferably something enjoyable as you mull these things over for a few days. Relax into your daily processes while your subconscious slowly sorts out the pieces.

* * *

I Remember . . . My Fear of Losing Him

I remember being afraid to let go of him, even though he had become a monster, who hit me and ran around on me—to name only a few problems. I just knew that if I let go some other woman would swoop him up, and that he'd then settle down and become a sweet and wonderful guy. I was afraid that he'd finally control his drinking, make a wonderful home for her, and I would have lost him—this incredible man—forever.

Well, in the twenty years since, I've discovered that not a single one of the undisclosed number of men I had loved and left had changed—those I knew of were still Horse's Butts. Or dead. Certainly none of them had changed enough that I could bear seeing them again, much less live with them. Oh, by the way—their lack of change was true even with all those new partners.

I Also Remember . . .

A couple of years ago (some 50 years after my divorce from him), an ex-husband, father of my four sons, called me—out of the blue. Hadn't heard from him in 30 years—and had never received even a dollar in child support from him.

Because this man had been extremely violent, I long ago determined to avoid any contact with him and gladly sacrificed the pittance he would have paid for child support to hide from and avoid him. Nevertheless, when he called I was curious on the chance he was calling about something important to do with the boys, so I didn't hang up immediately, my reflex response.

"Why are you calling me?" I said, with no friendly tone.

"Oh, there's no problem," he said. "I'm just checking up to see how you are doing."

"Huh," I said. I was surprised, shocked, and in the clutches of a minor Brain Freeze because of it.

"I'm rather busy and need to Move Along," I finally said.

"I just wanted to talk about the old times," he said, the nice guy plea in his voice, a tone that I remembered well although it had been nearly 50 years since I had heard it.

I'm sure my next words sprang from years of practice because they came automatically. I was getting practice through the years too every time I coached a woman on memorizing and using similar words:

"Bubba (we're Southern remember), I really don't want to talk with you. If I liked you at all, I'd probably still be married to you. I don't want to talk to you and I don't want you ever to call me again."

"But baby," he sprang back, with that same old wounded puppy whine in his voice, "what's wrong with talking? We're both older now, it's all in the past, why can't we just talk? I just wanted to talk about all the good times we had together."

I was dumbfounded. Speechless.

What did he just say? "All the good times"?

The surprise and perhaps a tinge of rage created a lot of energy to bolster my reply. I became extremely assertive (well, perhaps a bit aggressive) when I reflexively said, "Good times? Are you nuts? What do you mean 'good times'? I don't remember any good times!

"I do remember that you cheated on me so many times that I can't remember how many. I do remember that you lied to me even more times. I remember that you wouldn't work, that you took all the money that I made. I remember how awful you talked to me, the names you called me, the hateful things you said to me and told other people about me. And I remember that you hit me—a lot, and sometimes beat me horribly. I remember . . . ." And now he was shouting, interrupting me.

"See how you are?" his voice now nasal, strident. The old blaming tone I also remembered so well.

Then he launched the attack (his old trick that used to cower me because I felt so inadequate, and so aware of the power of his fists.)

"You know," he said then, with more stridency, "this is what was always wrong with you!" A breath: "You're so negative!"

I was flabbergasted, but only for a moment. Because of years of learning and practicing assertiveness, developing a lovely self-esteem and a sense of my goodness and value, as well as a lot of self-confidence, I blurted out, "Good-bye. Don't **ever** call me again." Click.

(Later, my youngest son told me his dad had called him and asked what in the world was wrong with his mother. He complained that I had been nasty to him! Can you believe it! Oh, yeah—I forgot—you can.)

This man, who, all those years ago I was so afraid to let go of because he might change—turn it all around and become wonderful and I'd miss out on it—had not changed one whit in the nearly half-century since then.

He still used the old switch-and-attack tricks that he used back then, when they worked so well for him.

More proof that he had not changed is the fact that he called me at all. After all these years (and several additional marriages that also failed for the same reasons ours did) he was still in total denial of his bad behavior.

Don't even think of pointing out the harm he inflicted on me *(and his four sons) in the doing, he was still jumping up to blame me for the problem!*

Sheesh.

So much for my fear of losing him because he might change and become wonderful and some other woman would get all that good stuff! Hah!

* * *

Another Kind of Story

A couple of buddies, Tom and Chet, over-drinkers both—finally found recovery after many, many tries.

Their drinking buddy George didn't make it though. He continued to drink and deteriorate.

The first couple of years, Tom and Chet tried to get George to come with them to the recovery program that was working so well for them, but he staunchly refused. "I don't need that!" he'd say, "I'm not that bad."

His life being unattractive to his friends, and theirs to him, they soon drifted apart.

About a year later, Chet saw George's obituary in the paper. Dismayed, he called Tom. They went sadly to the funeral home, where they found out that George had died of liver failure (the most common killer of over-drinkers who don't kill themselves in accidents or suicide before the liver goes).

They determined (correctly) that Chet's drinking had killed him and they felt really bad about it.

The next day, after the funeral service, Tom and Chet offered their sympathy to George's wife. They told her that George had been a good friend and asked if there was anything they could do to help her. She said no.

Then Tom asked if George had ever gone into any kind of alcohol treatment.

Aghast, George's wife drew back and, looking down her nose at them, said, "What do you mean? He wasn't *that* bad!"

Hmm.

He wasn't *that* bad?
He was only dead!

This, my lovelies, is a perfect example of that thing we will call "partner denial."

* * *

Chapter 6

Where you get a glimpse inside his head

Denial: Who's He Fooling?

Isn't "Denial" Actually Just Lying?
That's a question I get at almost every talk.
My answer is—Yes.
And no.
Yes, he definitely will lie. At some point he will be able to lie and be completely aware that he is lying, yet not blink an eye. He also can lie without being aware that what he's saying is a lie.

The mental gymnastic called "denial" differs from other psychological states because it requires denying something you have to be aware for your subconscious to know you need to lie.

He just doesn't always know for sure that he's lying. Or he knows he's lying, even a little bit, but he has justified it in his own mind because he thinks (erroneously) that his case is special. (All these are reasons why you need never again dig at him for the truth or challenge him about it. Just nod and go do something fun.)

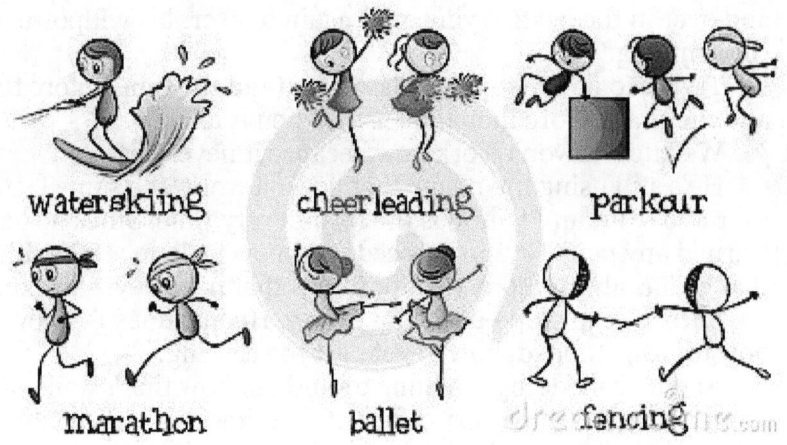

Frequently he believes his own lies; the more often he's told one, the more he believes it himself. That's when it comes out sounding more sincere: "I only had a couple." Because he believes this, since he has figured out that having more than a couple still covers "having a couple."

I Remember

Although I figured that out too. If I've had a six pack, I had to have had "a couple," so I could say that; it was kind of true.

* * *

Denial and Lying

"Gee, I guess I passed out in the car."
"I swear I'll stop—I mean it!"

And he may mean it--when he says it. In that case it may not be a total lie. But here's the problem: He doesn't have a clue *how* to do what he's swearing to. He doesn't know how to stop—and stay stopped. Even if he believes what he's saying, you will know better. He cannot get better if he doesn't learn how to do something different.

If he has not looked for or received any help or guidance, there is no way he can do what he says—he cannot stop and stay stopped. All he has available are the same things he's used over and over in the past. Trying once again to exert his willpower on the drinking.

Trying to do it like he did last time (and the time before that and the time before that and . . . .) When it failed.

We know it won't work now because it never has.

He's still using the recipe that doesn't work, the same tactics over and over, and failure is the result every time. Since he hasn't learned any *new* ways to succeed, we know he'll do all the things that he has always done to quit, things that have never worked.

Sure, he can stop—any drinker *can*. He just doesn't know how to *stay* stopped, how to get past the craving.

And he isn't doing anything to find out how that's done. If he doesn't do something very different this time, his well-meant attempt won't work . Again. And he just doesn't see or accept it.

Something new and different: People almost never are able to do it on their own. Those that I've followed up turned out to be doing many of the things for one reason or another that the successful methods of recovery (the greatest success, which is still less than 10 percent) teach.

Research shows that the only effective way to beat this problem is with a group—a group of people who drank like he has been drinking, and who all are holding each other up while they learn new tricks to beat the Devil. Doing it on one's own is a wash even before it starts. He's relying on what he already know—which has never been enough.

A special church group, an Alcoholics Anonymous group, a group at the VA, a group in a therapist's office. Those are some of the choices open to him. But always it must be a group—to succeed. I've heard people say someone did it without all that; they just went to church. That's a group.

Only a group works for recovery. Any kind of recovery. He needs at least one other person who is very like himself. This is the magic that works. The more men much like him and working for the same things, the more likely he will make it.

As a group, men much like him open up and talk about some of the things they've gotten into, and about how they can't seem to stay quit. They finally find out that they aren't the only ones with all this failure.

He'll hear such things as this: "I can't get by that desire for a drink that gradually swallows me completely." Then he'll hear several group members share some of the things that are working for them. He begins to see that it is absolutely possible for him to stay quit. After all, these other guys are doing it.

What Does His Denial Cost?

His denial is expensive; it costs him dearly. And it costs *you* dearly.

It will eventually cost him his life—or what passes for a life. In far too many cases, it costs his partner's life too, even if it only robs her of her health or mental stability, it's a loss of her life.

His denial that there's anything wrong with him while throwing all blame elsewhere, frequently on you, has cost you much of your self-confidence (which affects everything you do). He is totally invested in making you feel less than him, and it works in almost every case. This causes you to devalue yourself, to mistrust your own judgement, to feel stupid. Or crazy.

Causing you to doubt yourself is one of the worst mental and emotional damages to arise from your relationship with this man. He may be a sorry excuse for a man, or he may be a man who started out good and still has some of that (somewhere in there), but by Middle Stage his deepening need to protect his drinking has become more powerful than his love or respect for others. He will eventually deny love in order to maintain his suicidal drive to drink as he wishes. If (when) you leave him, he'll tell himself he doesn't love you, or never has.

Your cure? Accept that he has a damaged and impaired brain. This means that what he thinks is always suspect. His opinion is not enough to prove anything is true. He is not in his right mind, no matter how convincing he seems. (To be sure, he even believes most of his junk himself—further proof of his diminished intelligence.)

He believes that telling you half-truths is telling you the truth, or most of the truth. To protect his ability to drink without interference, he will both consciously and subconsciously shape his stories to fit that purpose. For him, being able to drink is survival, if only mental and emotional; anything he perceives as threatening results in reactions only slightly less than if you came at him with an axe.

His responses to threats to both ego and drinking are not intelligent responses; they are driven by his primal brain, sometimes referred to as the "reptile brain." (A snake brain.) His reflex reactions have no hidden meaning. You just don't understand what's happening. He reacts this way because his deepest self believes he must be able to drink when he needs to. Considering having that blocked creates a snake-brain-deep panic. At gut level, certainly not intellectual level, he reflexively responds to any threat to his ego or his drinking as he would to a threat on his life.

No, his intelligent mind will know better, at least until Middle-Middle Stage, but by then his intelligent mind is no longer running the show. His snake-brain is. Your proof of that? He can't stay quit! Intelligently, he has clarity and often the strong desire to stop and not to hurt others; but that deep, deep level, nestled in the heart of his survival instinct, is wired (as in all people) to override all else when there's a conflict of thinking. And it does.

Your cost is to live in chaos, to doubt yourself, to lose your self-confidence, your happiness, to live your life in segments around crises he creates. That, beautiful girl, is not living. That cost is too great to ignore. It's why his problem can kill you before it kills him.

So, all that said, let's proceed with learning as much as you can about what's going on in his head. You can start by considering what kind of a brain can fool itself about itself, the personality that fools itself about itself. If it weren't so destructive to his woman you could just call it pathetic. But it's worse than that; it does harm.

* * *

He Really, Really Wants to Think That He's not as Bad As Other Over-Drinkers

Over-drinkers work very hard to feel and appear unique, to convince others that their case is special, that they are not like regular "drunks." To do this they must bat down or ignore any reality that doesn't line up with their take on it.

Denial tactics include "shading" truth, just slightly bending it so it stays fairly close to truth; and then there are the outright lies, but usually only "when I was desperate".(they tell themselves). The purpose of these mental acrobats is just one thing: to protect the image they need to project. That image they are determined to project is that they are above reproach and, therefore, can't have a problem. A gentle, caring girl will get run over every time with this tactic.

Over-drinkers will continue to protect this flimsy image, even when it's already been shattered. They do it both consciously and unconsciously—and at almost any cost.

He lies sometimes because he really can't remember the truth, at least not much of it. His well-meaning denial system may be hiding it even from himself. In this form of truth-bending, he fills in the blanks with something keeping him as close to appearing wonderful as he can manage. These are where you can get a rage in return for asking the simplest question about what he's just said.

He also can tell lies when he knows he's lying, which is the most frequent kind, but fortunately, they are usually the easiest to detect. Just two or many tip-offs are an artificial casualness, or avoiding eye contact. A man who will look you in the eye while he lies to you is a dangerous man. You do well to disbelieve anything he says.

So he can tell lies that he knows are lies, and he can tell lies that he's not sure whether they are lies or not, and he can tell lies that he actually doesn't know are lies.

So how in the world can you really know when he's telling the truth?

Here's a hint on that topic; it comes from recovery groups:

Some one in a recovery group says: "Know how to tell when a drinker is lying?"

And someone else will answer, "Yes, it's when his lips are moving!"

Does that seem cruel? Yet it's based on the truths you just read about how he can lie. His subconscious doesn't have the full picture and the rest of his brain is not equipped to straighten it all out.

All recovering people, the truly recovering, find this conversation to be quite funny and there is much laughter every time it comes up. (An over-drinker who is getting honest enough with himself to admit he has been a flagrant liar just may have a chance to be one of those 10 percent who make it.) The one who staunchly denies he's lied has no chance—until that changes.

Here's how it works: Whenever he gets in a fix, the first thing he does is run the facts of the event over and over in his head, searching for a loophole, one he can stretch around reality enough to slip through without having to be responsible for his behavior.

He also searches for where someone has done something he

can convince you was unjust, so that he, understandably, got drunk and did whatever it is he's covering up. If he can't find that loophole, he can invent one. And the primary purpose of the finished product is to removes any shadow appearing imperfect.

Why does he do that? Right—he does it because it works so well.

Sometimes he even convinces himself that he's without blame! Sometimes, like when he's had two or more drinks, he believes he's the blooming Man of The Year.

Knowing all this benefits you because it shows that your misery is wasted, twisting your brain trying to figure out if he's telling the truth. Stop knotting yourself up trying to prove it one way or the other. He believes his entire life depends on people believing what he says, and you are looking for a truth you're not all that sure you want—a sure recipe for confusion.

Quit second-guessing his stories. It is making you old before your time. Go find something fun to do.

Work on your dreams list or a plan for fulfilling one Work on what is the next step to move you closer to your desire.

Denial: Like with other areas of a drinker's life, love has nothing to do with it. Not how much he loves you and not how much you love him. For him, it's all and only about not letting anybody know what's really going on, which proves a part of him already knows he's in real trouble.

His denial isn't about loving you or anybody else; it's about his survival (and his deepest heart believes he cannot survive mentally, or won't want to, if he can't drink when he wants/needs it.)

Alcohol can shut down brain cells in his short-term memory, so that he has no memory of events during a period of time, although it's rare that there's a total shutdown. (He may claim it is, but it isn't. Throughout the next day or so, he'll get flashes of the truth and those memories will be quite disgusting to him—which is precisely why his subconscious shoved them into his denial box. The glimpses of memory that work their way through, he'll try to shut down, squish up his eyes and shudder—I call them memory shorts, trailers—accurate memory that he doesn't want to face. And he does not want to see the whole movie.

(One excellent example of what he calls "shading" the truth is saying he has had "a couple" of drinks.)

Flash! He does not feel like he's lying. He *has* had "a couple." (And then some.)

The brain cells required for working with truth are dozing off.

His thinking and behavior get still weirder as his need increases to hide things he doesn't want others to know.

By now, you likely understand why I urge you to stop digging for "truth." First of all, if it's a nasty truth don't jump in—like jumping in a cesspool where you may drown. Also, you will rarely ever know if what you finally get to is the real truth. You will have lost much time and energy and still be left bleeding emotionally.

Perhaps the most harmful result of digging for his truth is that it can rapidly becomes an obsession; because it has to do with your wiring—your nest—it can eat you alive, consume you, rob you of time and energy you could spend on getting a fulfilling life. Or just getting a life. And it can fire up some of your own crazy behavior. (Besides, when you grill him or dig at the truth, it only makes him work harder to improve his lying.) And never, ever let that Crazy Adult mixed into your subconscious beat you by reminding you over and over of the ugly thing he has done or said. When that starts, it is coming from your Wounded Inner Child, and she is not well enough yet to let her take over your thinking. Gently tell her that you think she's beautiful and good, and help her let go of the memory of his ugly deeds or words.

You don't deny they occurred; you just refuse to smother yourself in them. Your conscious mind makes a healthy decision in its job of protecting you.

(Note: "Letting Go" that wonderful Alanon trick, is worth getting yourself over to them and learning. Once you understand it, it will help tremendously in these situations.)

The fact that he's in denial of any form is an admission of guilt. A person only denies things he/she thinks are bad. With the chances of his lying being so very high, if you wonder whether he's being truthful, your doubt is enough to assume that most of what he says is skirting the truth. Don't push—now. There may come a time when you will get more truth, but it's not now. All you can get now is more hostility—and you've had quite enough of that, thank you.

If you have decided it's best for you to stay with him, you will have to learn this trick. The longer you put that off, the greater will be your pain. It will destroy you, not him.

Letting Go comes easier when you Move Along. Keep up your pace and go do something fun, reminding yourself on the way that you decided to stay with this man and this for a very good reason. And you are free to reassess that position at any time.

He can be unpredictable: Sometimes it's "God help anyone who sees things differently than what he's saying." Other times, he can collapse in regretful sobs. What he actually thinks and feels is all of that and if you actually get to the bottom of it, it turns out to be a mish-mash, mixed with a kind of nutsy logic that almost, almost makes sense and can leave you in worse shape than when you started your inquiry. He will consciously and unconsciously play on your sympathies or other emotions (such as anger where if he gets you there, he can keep pushing until you pop off and then he can blame everything on your blow-up. Slam!

By the way, don't make any threat about leaving or whatever else you might think of to threaten. Never threaten anything unless you are already secure in a plan for safe separating. The time will eventually come, may already be here, when an "or else," results in his choosing the "or else."

People Are Hard-Wired for Denial
"Denial" is a psychological, sometimes subconscious, mechanism that lies below their level of everyday consciousness. "Denial" in healthy people is intended to protect us after a severe emotional blow, a numbing, shielding us briefly from the pain. It's designed to work for a short while., which is how many get into trouble: When the numb brain begins to wake up, one who still has no way to cope with the reality will be forced to find another pain-killer--alcohol or drugs, gambling and sex, anything to take over their minds to keep their brains so dull or busy that they don't feel.

Denial, functioning as intended, is a tremendous tool for mental and emotional survival. It temporarily numbs emotions so you can continue functioning in life-sustaining ways. You aren't slammed with massive pain all at once. But, as with other remarkable wiring intended to aid mankind, used incorrectly, it can destroy us.

Psych Note: Being in even minor denial indicates that he is

> already in big trouble with his drinking. It is sufficient proof that his drinking has become a problem that is big enough for part of him to want to hide the truth.
>
> Why does he do that? So he doesn't have to change and give up something that feels so very good to him, that has become so very necessary to him.
>
> It has very little to do with you; he's hiding the truth even from himself.

(Note: To probe for a patient's veracity, a professional needs only to ask family members who live with or near him about his drinking, then compare their answers to his. Discrepancy indicates denial, which indicates that part of him knows full well that he is drinking too much.)

    As drinking progresses, denial progresses. At the same time he knows at some level that he is selling off his health, his life, his family, everything good and holy in his life to continue getting the feeling he needs from alcohol, The belief that alcohol is necessary goes so deep, is so strong, that only a handful will ever escape either the belief or the alcohol. The lie, that he needs to drink when he needs to, always pulls him back to the lover who, like a black widow, will kill him in return. Part of a drinker knows that, yet goes on, making continuing in the face of all the information out there today a measure of how total is his mental fixation.)

    Most over-drinkers will maintain until the Late or End stages that their drinking isn't as bad as other people who drink too much. Maintaining that his case is different, he believes that his drinking is a special case. Understanding this sheds light on most of his behavior. Maintaining his illusion that he is superior compels him to make you look and feel like the Dummy Witch of the West.

    He thinks dummies aren't qualified to question him, or point out any flaw. His need to appear above reproach is why he tears down others. His drive to appear unassailable seems to know no bounds. And it usually works—right up to the Late Stage. Until then, when his act is assailed, he can get very ugly. If he allows you (or anyone) to think you know better than he it would mean he needed to bow to their assessments of his drinking and behavior. Rest assured, he will do almost anything to avoid that. That's because he knows others will expect or demand that he stop drinking. And he knows he can't.

When he's puffing up, criticizing you, calling you names, putting you down, that's Really Good News—from now on! That proves he is aware he has a need whose fulfillment he must protect at any cost. It proves that You Are Right!

All that ugliness he slings out when his perfection is questioned IS NOT about you. While you, like all the rest of humanity, are not a saint, he (or anyone) can always find something about you, present or past, to point at and try to beat you down with. To pretend they are superior because you have a flaw! You now cease to believe this screwy thinking.

* * *

> **Psych Note:** In the past you've labored at correcting all the imperfections in yourself that he points out, at first to make him happy, later, just to avoid his attacks. But he needs to make you feel inferior so he can stay in control. Your mental salvation: His verbal attacks just aren't about you!
>
> His finding flaws in you is all about the need he has to feel superior, above reproach. It's not about your mistake or imperfection. It's about his need to look good; he believes he can do that by making someone else look bad. He can hook you because of your own underlying belief that you aren't "good enough."

Eventually the drinker needs to feel superior to everyone, including doctors and other professionals (especially those who suggest he needs to do something about his drinking!). When he starts criticizing you or anyone else, recall that he thinks that by pointing out their flaws, it makes them less credible in their judgements of him and, even better, it makes him look superior. (A part of him knows that he isn't superior, else he wouldn't work so hard to make the point.) The added payoff for him is that people come to avoid finding fault with him just because he responds with such vitriol (which was his intent all along).

One of his favorite tricks is defending himself and his drinking with comparisons, trying to make himself look good: "Well, I may drink, but I'm not as bad as old Herman down the street." And, "Me? A drunk? You wanna see a drunk? Go down to old Herman's house. Now that's a drunk!" And all of this comes from your trying to talk to him about coming home last night and passing out in the yard, then puking on the porch this morning when the neighbors were watching. He compares his "sin" to one that he thinks is worse--an effort to make his sin appear small. He thinks that because Ted Bundy murdered lots of people, and he only drinks a bit and is a Horse's Butt, it means he's wonderful!" Snake brain.

He has probably already one-upped you; it would go like this: "Oh, yeah? You think I'm bad? Well, at least I'm not out chasing women like Old Don! You ought to be grateful for that—and quit complaining about all this baloney." (Never mind that you know he hasn't been able to function sexually for quite a while, which may be why he doesn't chase now that his priorities and self-control are so fouled up.)

No, baby, it's not you with the mental problem.

> **Psych Note:** He is driven to make sure others believe his "stuff." He works at getting them to see things his way.
>
> This reminds me of a French term in psychology—"folies a deux," which translates as "the folly of two."
>
> Folies a deux describes a situation where one person convinces another that a fantasy, even a hallucination, is real. (This would occur when a patient comes in and tells his therapist that aliens are trying to take over his head and describes the way they do it so well that the therapist wonders if his head is safe from head invasion.)
>
> When you even half-believe his tales, it's folies a deux.
>
> **Beware of folies a deux!**

Research shows that no one is much better than anyone else at detecting lies. The most wonderful FBI agent is barely any better at detecting lies than you or me. Most drinkers's women believe they know when their guy is lying, and they certainly recognize a blatant lie; but the mass of lies, many of them important, may be slipping under the wire. To improve your accuracy, judge his truthfulness by your gut: If you think he's ling, he likely is.

He Believes His Excuses Prove He's Unique

An over-drinker collects bad experiences like Scrooge McDuck hoards money. The over-drinker treasures his bad experiences! Saves them up. To him they are gold—these examples of how others have mistreated him or his undeserved bad luck are stored in his vault, handy, where he can grab one in a flash when needed. (Mind you, he stores these events in a memory that can't remember what time he said he'd be home.)

Frequently over-drinkers have had many bad life experiences. Many, however, are the result of something to do with his drinking. He well may have had a hard childhood or other great difficulty. Being as you have the softest heart of almost any personality type, you must accept some reality here: Bad things happen to everyone—but only some of them think they excuse bad behavior.

Reality: Only a few people who have bad experiences use them to excuse over-drinking or bad behavior.

Most people buy right into his excuses for over-drinking because they believe that people over-drink because something bad happened to them.

But we know that's not true.

Billions of people have suffered terrible, horrible things, yet only some of them use that as an excuse to drink or behave badly.

(Being able to conjure up "reasons" for over-drinking is important to an over-drinker; he puts great amounts of mental energy into it. He can't allow anyone to think he's just a drunk! Heaven forbid.)

Now that you better understand the crazy thinking involved, you are going to be harder to manipulate. Of course, that means he likely will push a little harder—trying everything he has ever used to get you riled up, or to fool you. Knowing now what's really going on, I'm sure you will see to it that his dirty tricks no longer work.

A suggested response to a tale of woe:

"Gee, I'm so sorry you had a bad day, dear, but what does that have to do with being late and drunk?"

Then Stretchy-Lip him and a Move Along.

He is capable of defending his twisted tales to the death, which is why you don't need to spend any more energy on this. The truth that he hides from is that he needs to drink, and needs it more than just about anything. Look at the things he loses or gives up on his way down: Friends, family, his health, finances, his sanity, his self-respect, you.

While over-drinkers sometimes admit, in self-pity or remorse, that they have a problem, it's usually when they are very drunk—or when trying to placate you. The next day you tell him what he said—"You said you've got a drinking problem; let's do something about it," he flares up and goes on the attack, or says, "Aw—I was drunk when I said that!" So much for protecting his superiority.

When less than falling-down drunk, the over-drinker can say: "Yeah, I know I probably drink more than I should. But what the heck! (Big grin.) We all have to go sometime! Ha-ha."

That's Denial.

What can you do about his weird affliction? Right—Nothing! Stretchy-Lip him and Move Along.

(Note: Don't feel guilty for doubting him. To doubt him, beyond the Early Middle Stage demonstrates your sanity. And you don't have to tell him about your doubt to have it.)

If an over-drinker is unable to distinguish between his own lies and the truth, how in the world can you expect to?

Okay, it's time to pick up another new trick, four easy steps that promise you greater peace of mind:

The "Plan B" Trick

1. You no longer let any of your plans (or your mental-emotional stability) depend on his promises or agreements.

2. You never again worry about whether he will do what he says. Assume there's a good chance he won't and fall back on another method.

3. Develop and use Plan B. Forget relying on him and live longer. And less stressed.

You are coming to accept that he is less reliable now—and the next step is to realize it has little or no relationship to how much he loves you. His unreliability has nothing at all to do with love. It has to do with twisted brain wiring and missing brain cells.

Having a Plan B in the background most of the time means

you will quickly notice your stress level dropping. This often coincides with catching yourself smiling more.

(I know, having a Plan B is not do-able all the time, so just do the best you can at any given moment.) Plan B is a wonderful way to take care of yourself (and your children if you have children). With a Plan B in the backstage area, you always have a fallback when he falls out, and that cushions your fall when he fails to do what he should do. It does put more work on you, just setting up alternate arrangements you can switch to; you will soon find it is well worth the effort for the peace of mind it gives you. Just knowing you have that cushion sweeps away stress around any event.

Example of a Plan B: He says he'll pick up Johnny's birthday cake on the way home that evening. Your Plan B is to check with the bakery and have someone in the background who has agreed to go for it if needed. Use a bakery near home so you can shoot out and get it if need be.

Plan B, Another Example: Say you've separated, and he says he'll pick up little Johnny Saturday at 4:00 o'clock. You have something or someone else lined up in the wings for both you and Johnny to enjoy should the drinker fail to follow through. This way, it's win-win. Better still, you are now a big girl! Taking your own mental wellbeing in hand, taking care of yourself.

The only difference is that you no longer let yourself believe he's reliable: Now you know that it's always a 50-50 shot—either he will or won't; so you are ready for either.

Likewise, your emotional happiness and mental stability can't depend on what someone with a broken mind says or does. You will no longer allow him to be the keeper of your happiness, and now you cease allowing him to be in control of your stress level whenever possible.

Does this new perspective break your trust bond? Yes—but, by now it's already been broken for a while.

Examples of DENIAL

"Yeah, I know that <u>sometimes</u> I can be a Horse's Butt."

(This technique: <u>Minimizing</u>, making it sound less than it really is; avoiding the full truth.)

So he can appear truthful (sometimes because he believes his own stories), humble (one of his really good tricks), but in truth, his "admissions" are probably always under-reported by now. He has so much more need to protect his ability to drink and behave as he wishes without question. His primary goal by Mid-Middle Stage: staying free to drink as he wishes.

He also minimizes the impact of his bad behavior on others, to them, to others, and to himself. He's seeking to escape close examination.

Are You in Denial Too?

One up-side of over-drinkers all becoming more and more alike as they disintegrate is that, after the Early Stages, their behavior becomes pretty predictable.

You want to think he won't do things other over-drinkers do, or at least not as bad as others do, but that want has the power to make you believe the lie. And that is firing up your own Denial system. Take some time to explore what your fears are about acknowledging that he is likely to begin moving faster toward the worst stages.

Getting them on paper allows you to ponder ways to avoid or cope with what may be coming.

Your denial is trying to protect you from the stressor of all the bad things that can happen is he gets worse. But continuing living on a hope that has virtually no chance of being fact, is guaranteed to bring you an rougher road than what you are fearing. Whether it's difficult to separate, break up your home, or simply face the death of your dream of love—do not blind yourself to the possibilities and begin planning for them.

Once you pry out exactly what you fear may happen to you, you move ahead. A good counselor can be very helpful in this. One or two sessions should be enough. (Be sure to find out whether the licensed, female counselor you choose is willing to do what we call "short-term therapy." This is therapy that focuses on a single point. It does very little digging into the past. And it doesn't aim to fix your life, only assist you to make a difficult life choice.

* * *

List some of the things you fear might happen if you accept the fact that he's really that bad:

1. _____

2. _____

3. _____

Your fear of these very outcomes are what causes your denial. Seeing and accepting the truth may mean you'll face something that appears too difficult for you. But don't sell yourself short, girl. You're much tougher than you may sometimes believe. (Look at what you've already endured! Yeah, you're spunky.)

Psych Note: Your buttons can only be pushed if you believe two things:

1. The caustic remark made about you has even a smidgen of truth, (doesn't have to be true, just that you *believe* it is) and

2. You believe it's important to be totally free of that negative element because you believe it would detract from you or harm you in some way.

(Yet another set of buttons are pushed if you believe someone else believes the negative remark is true.)

Recovery: The very first step is to accept the fact that you really are only human. (By the way, after a year or so of doing this, it becomes a comfortable part of your thinking. Just keep it up and you'll be free of the pain that negative judgements of you used to produce.) It's more difficult for most of you than for other people—mostly because you have been criticized (perhaps all your life), an element that I have found to be true in almost every case of "co-dependency" or being a drinker's woman.

At first, admitting to yourself that you're not perfect can feel like a kind of death mixed in with the surety that no one will ever love you because you're not good enough ("good enough" meaning "perfect" to you).

Still, you're both spunky *and* smart. You know at some level that there is no such thing as a perfect person, that you, with all

> the other five billion people in the world, are all flawed some way. Getting honest with yourself now about this very thing, the impossibility of ever becoming perfect **and** that being perfect is a necessary quality to be loved.
>
> Pondering these ideas, where they came from in you, and how they have caused you pain for your entire life, as well as how ridiculous they are, leads to your gradually beginning to give yourself some slack.
>
> Here's your goal: Start immediately working on being as gentle on yourself as you tend to be to most others.
>
> Being human means you are always subject to making a mistake, to being wrong, as is everyone else on the planet. Bring that reality to mind as often as you can. Be as gentle with yourself as you would be to a dear friend. Getting comfortable with the reality of not being perfect goes hand in hand with giving yourself credit for your good traits and qualities. Myself, I figure that I may not be a good cook, but I'm a great grandmother! And I am good-hearted, have a great sense of humor, and do lots of nice things for other people, so I'm sorry you think I fall short in my housekeeping or cooking. After a few years of chewing on these ideas, they are a solid part of me—and of every other woman who has grabbed hold of them and gone for the gold.

Nobody and no-thing is perfect! That means anyone can find a flaw in anyone or anything. Trouble is that some people think that ability makes them superior. Oh, well. We just Stretchy-Lip them, and Move Along.

You never *will* be perfect. You've been caught up in trying to be because you believed that others's attitude and bad treatment of you have been because you have flaws, you aren't perfect. Let me remind you that most of you have been so deprived of real love, not the kind you had to earn but from someone who focused on your beauty and loved you for it.

Your reflex, when criticized, has been to turn yourself inside out in search of exactly what is wrong and how to make it perfect.

Give it up, child. Give the world your smile and your best traits! It is more than adequate. You are wonderful and special— but not perfect! Thank goodness!

Now we come to the trick that has the power to truly set you free from this feared, hated occurrence—when someone finds you lacking: The Freedom Trick.

> **The Freedom Trick**
>
> 1. Acknowledging an imperfection sets you free! Admit you may have made a mistake or have been wrong. Big deal! "Oh, I was wrong about that!" Stretch 'Em.
>
> 2. Correct any true error by thinking how you might do the same thing better next time it comes up, then
>
> 3. Let go! Go do something fun.

The idea that being perfect is what will get you the love you hunger for is deeply rooted. And it's totally wrong. For many of you, it goes all the way back, perhaps to an infant who was screamed at or rejected for crying to have its needs met. That baby would have learned very, very early that it needed to ignore its vital needs if it was to be cared for at all. Only the very lucky got love too.

* * *

What happens to you when he criticizes you?
What he is demanding is that you do or be what his broken mind wants you to be at that moment. There is little or no room left for being who you truly are.
And where did he learn how to punch your buttons? Oh yes! You taught him that! He learned by noticing your responses to things he said or did, then when he wanted any specific reaction, he knew exactly what to do.
In the past, when something tipped over your apple barrel, he took note of it. Once you understand that much of what he does is to get your goat, if only to prove he is a superior person, recall that he learned how directly from you! Once you realize this, you're on your way to breaking up his game.
From this moment, to the best of your ability at any given moment, you are going to make a screeching stop to responding to him in any of your old ways. You will overwork Stretchy-Lip and Move Along instead.

The fastest way to stop having your buttons pushed is to start freezing when you feel a reaction coming on—or recognize that you're in the middle of it. Just stop. You can Stretch 'Em at any time and break up your own unwanted response. Then you Move Along.

Whatever you do now blows a hole in his method. All you need do is repeat your new response a time or two, and most of his get-your-goat tricks will stop. Except once in a great while, he'll test you. If he doesn't get the reward he is after, it causes his subconscious to begin erasing that act from his tool box.

It's the process of breaking any habit. Make it stop being rewarding!

Before he gives up, however, he may at first think you just didn't hear him, so what will he do? Yes—he'll repeat what he said, probably louder. Perhaps he'll say something worse. But you're onto him now. You don't let on at all that it bothers you. Stretch 'Em.

Move Along.

When he upsets you, Stretch 'Em and Move Along. Better this than getting into something that will cost plenty and accomplish nothing.

Remember that whatever you used to do when you were upset is what he's trying to make you do again! Sometimes he may even do these things subconsciously, but that doesn't change his purpose. (If he's a true psychopath, of course, he consciously works at pushing your buttons. If this is your situation, you may not be safe. He will not (cannot) change. It's time to reconsider your living situation. If you aren't quite sure what a "psychopath" is, I urge you to look it up; it's a very serious mental disorder, and often dangerous to those around one.

A Biggie—The Southern Girl's Trick: Yes, Honey

Even though you are powerless against the mental mechanisms driving him, simple tricks will save you aggravation, frustration, even emotional pain. A tactic that has worked beautifully for us Southern girls for 100 years is a simple three-step trick that I call

The "Yes-Honey" Trick

1. He says something ridiculous, outrageous, or untrue; you catch yourself coming back to argue the point or defend yourself:

you Clamp 'Em! Clamp jaws and lips.

2. Auto-Stretchy-Lip (with one addition): You partially release your jaws to slip out, "Okay, honey." Not a word more! Say it as if agreeing with whatever he is saying.

3. Now Clamp 'Em! again and Move Along.

Some have said they feel guilty about this trick, dishonest. Well maybe, from a certain viewpoint. But the viewpoint *we* are going to take is that you aren't actually agreeing to what he says, only signaling that you hear him.
At first, your "Yes, Honey" may create surprise; expect that.
It may bring that brief brain stall (always obvious on his face and so enjoyable to behold). Or he may be sarcastic: "What? You're just going to agree?" Or, "Wait a minute. I'm not through."
No matter what he responds, you politely respond: "Okay, just a minute—I've got to run to the bathroom"—or some other undeniable emergency.
Smoke!
Doorbell!
Phone!
Baby crying!
Oops! Started my period!

* * *

MASTERY

Pull out one or two points from this chapter that you want to absorb totally and rapidly and write them here.

1. _____

_____

2. _____

_____

Chapter 7

Where you
> Find out how to ease your discomfort and emotional pain
> Find out more of what's happening to you
> Get started fixing what you find!

Prince Being Beastly; How Fares Fair Princess?

Tell me three good things about yourself on the lines below. (Your good qualities, good traits, abilities and skills, and more about you that you know are good—No! Not Perfect! Just *Good*!). Include things you do well, your skills, talents, your thinking habits, even your attitudes. No! Not the kind that you practice 100 percent! Just those that you know are good things.

1. _____

2. _____

3. _____

Now list three more:

4. _____

5. _____

6. _____

Now just pull up one more. Take the time to copy these items, the good stuff about you, onto your Note pages in the back of the book. You know—repetition.

_____

I asked you to write this list for me. Next, I want you to take ownership of the list, of each of the qualities you listed, one by one. These are good things about *you,* *t*hings people who take the time can see (except maybe your thinking habits). When you are in doubt, recognize that you possess a quality if you have it to any extent. If you feel more honest about it, you can add something like a percentage by the item, but even Jesus wasn't perfect—in the eyes of those watching Him. Remember when He busted up the tables at the church? How about when He called the people giving him a hard time sons of vipers?

We all suffer from the limits of our given culture, judging ourselves by what the culture says "nice girls" do or don't do. Or don't do enough—which is usually your problem in judging yourself. Girl, sometimes the well runs dry and can only produce a half-bucket of water, but does that mean the well doesn't give water? Lighten up on yourself; if you have a *good* quality to any extent, I repeat, list it.

Later, likely not until the follow-up book to this one about curing your quirks, you are going to go deeper into this idea. I have discovered in my many years of experience with mental health that the qualities people judge as bad in themselves turn out to be only a lack or shortage of some good quality. If that's confusing, let it be for now. We'll go deeper later. Your next step here is building this material into your thinking, your mind, and by thinking about the list and the qualities often, that list will become part of your subconscious.

At that point, you will stop (or nearly stop) judging yourself negatively. You will recognize your true value, perhaps the reason you're on this planet.

Now read *aloud* each of the items you have listed. Think of ONE time when you demonstrated that quality. When you recall that reality, you must then admit to yourself that you actually have that quality—10 percent level or 99 percent, you own whatever it is.

Go down this entire list. It well may take you some time— certainly some quiet time. Your list is not a one-time adventure but is now becoming very much a part of your entire being, where one good quality in you recognizes that you have another, and another, and . . .

This exercise constitutes the packing material for a separate bag of tricks, the tricks that have the power to change your thinking from dark to light, morose to hopeful. You will use this special bag of tricks for stopping the jack hammer in your head when it cranks up trying to dig out something about you that you think is bad. It can shut that puppy right down, like magic.

In the process, your sense of yourself grows more strongly beautiful, until most of the time you are happy to be just who you are, pretty much just like you are.

This first exercise into the special bag is the heart of a gaggle of tricks to come, all of which will make use of these reminders of the *many* good things about you.

> **Psych Note:** One terribly destructive effect of criticism, whether from others or yourself (and these have nearly equal power to harm you), especially if you believe and dwell on your failure to be up to some particular standard (which your subconscious interprets as proving that you are inadequate), is to chop away, even erase a positive sense of self in the receiver.
>
> A deep well of painful experiences with critical people have shaped most of you into the perfect shape to fit a distorted judge. That personality element is strong in you, Luke—uh, I mean it's strong in you, else you could not have become wounded in this way. That personality element causes you to latch on to negative judgements in an attempt to make the bad thing go away.
>
> The learned way of grabbing onto any hint of a negative comment about yourself, believing it—even to a small extent—then obsessing on how to get rid of the trait supposedly earning the criticism. The result is that, due to the wounded sense of self and the sense of inadequacy, even inferiority, his woman doesn't believe, at the level where it counts, that she doesn't deserve any better. And can't do or get any better.
>
> That entire mess is fueled by the mass of unfulfilled emotional needs in the person who becomes the target of critical others.
>
> This beaten-down sense of self then becomes the major offender in creating a person who allows others to hurt them, not consciously, but through their learned way of accepting those negative judgements. Taking them to heart becomes the corrosive factor in breaking down a person's self-esteem, self-confidence, and positive sense of self.
>
> Sometimes, just understanding what has happened blasts people out of the pit of self-dissatisfaction, self-condemnation.

> A malnourished sense of self happens totally because deep down in the subconscious, if not their fully conscious mind, this person (likely you) believes she doesn't deserve the rewards of feeling pretty good about themselves. Of moving through their days knowing you have some good qualities that can brighten the world.
>
> That slashing away at any positive sense of self could be happening to you every time you take one nasty comment to heart.
>
> Baby, the negative judgements and comments floating around are just and only one person's opinion, and most people who voice negative judgements are simply not qualified to pass that judgement. Just because they say it, or think it, doesn't mean it's true, for Pete's sake.

I Remember

My mentor made me write lists. Several of which turned out to be the point where deep healing could begin. Off topic, this track brings to mind something that may show you that I've been way down on that low self-esteem ladder too.

My mentor told (ordered) me to list three things I was grateful for. I could not at the time. Everything I thought of turned out to fall short. My failure set him off: He launched out on one of his speeches. First, he lambasted me for not being grateful for anything, and when I played pitiful, like life was just too hard, he pointed out that I was finally free of alcohol—at least free for a day at a time.

That was a good start. Then he said that I should be grateful that I didn't go bald while I was over-drinking!

He was a bit strange, so I just waited to see what else he was working on. Of course, I had never even thought of being grateful for such a thing, or for losing hair and going bald due to stress, which I had suffered in spades for many years. He proceeded to educate me, pointing out a long list of little things I never think about being grateful for. Things like being grateful that gorillas and pythons don't roam free in my neighborhood, like that. But a few of the things he listed were solid; as I began to focus on them, I gained another tool for manipulating myself. Perhaps you can use this bit of my experience and the load of wisdom I gained thereby.

Turns out that alcohol is very hard on skin, and hair, and most over-drinkers start losing hair. I became immediately grateful. I did what he told me to and made my list. And don't give me credit for this surrender because, as it happened, it was "do it" or else he wouldn't mentor me anymore.

I tell you these things to be sure you know I'm not a golden girl, but that I am rather obstreperous (ha! look it up!). I'm thankful that quality in me has ramped down considerably. Not gone, but much reduced. My getting into difficult situations also ramped down about the same time.

Hmm—maybe there's a connection.

His guidance worked, by the way. I became truly grateful for my hair.

And that I don't have longer or thicker nose hair, which he added for good measure. I always have something to celebrate.

Making your list of good traits is a lot like making a list of things to be grateful for: It doesn't matter if the only good thing you can think of right now is that you haven't stolen chickens, wrung their heads off, and eaten them raw, it's still something good about you. *(My first item I could come up with was that I had never hurt an animal. Later I remembered that my father ordered me to sit behind the porch rail with a BB gun and shoot any dog that came to his garden. I did. Still breaks my heart to think about it. Even so, for a while it gave me one positive thing to drag my mind off what I thought were my many flaws.)*

And you too might add to your positives that you at least haven't lost all your hair, whether it fall out or you yanked it out yourself. Hair loss is a major result of long-term stress. And I'll bet that you have never set fire to a rhinoceros. Or to a Horse's Butt. In fact, you've refrained from doing most of the bad things you've wanted to do to him and I'm telling you that's a really big, good thing about you. (Have I already told you about a friend who confessed that she had once gone out in her yard and picked mushrooms from the grass, then made a pot of spaghetti sauce for his dinner? That she served them to him? She was terribly disappointed at the time that they apparently had no effect. Down the road, after they had tried her for murder, she'd have had a tad of disappointment anyway.)

Your very good quality of refraining is that, due to another good quality—that of being loathe to cause pain to others—you have refrained from doing some of the things that have come to mind at one time or another. Mind that I'm not saying you refrained *every* time, but even once is a star in your crown, especially when we recall the reasons such an idea ever popped into your mind.

So--Once you've listed the first six good things about you, post your list where you will see it daily. Noticing it even once a day will begin to strengthen and heal your wounded sense of your goodness and value; the list, posted, is also the most effective and fastest way to start erasing from your subconscious negative thoughts about yourself. (You want this because part of the reason you are stuck with this man is that you believe you're so flawed you can't do anything else.)

Your next reward that this practice automatically brings you is that items on the list of negatives about you begin to fade, then disappear.

The same tool will erase, swat away like slapping at wasps, the goofy and hateful things he can say about you. Having just three things good about you stuck fast in memory is your Golden Key to new freedom and the rebirth of your self-worth (and happiness).

Here's your first solid trick in your separate, The Pop Out and Replace Trick.

The Pop Out and Replace Trick.

1. **Catch it!** (Sound familiar?)Any time you find yourself thinking on something negative about yourself or that someone else has said about you, Catch It! And zip on to Step 2.

2. **Grab** *one* item from your list. Any item will do. (You will memorize the first three items, or the ones you think are your very best qualities.) This guarantees this step will flow rapidly, easily. (You only need one item, although the more the better, if you recall more than one at the moment, pull them into the mix too.)

3. **Focus** on a quality, see yourself being or doing that thing, realize you actually do have the quality.

4. **Substitute** the thought of that positive quality for the negative one circulating in there.

5. **Practice this:** "Hmph, I *could* be a little (whatever), but I *also* have some wonderful qualities! One of them is (whatever) fill in this blank with your good quality.

My experience with this trick was nothing short of miraculous, and almost every woman who has tried it has reported a wonderful experience with it.

I chose this form of talking to myself here: "I could have little talent as a cook, but I am good at seeing what others need at the moment, and helping them to get it. *(I love that quality in myself! Not surprisingly, it seems to erase from my brain a multitude of thoughts about shortcomings. This trick will do the same for you.)*

* * *

Stress Has Dangerous Effects

Now we come to the most dangerous effect an over-drinker has on his woman (short of violence and murder). His drinking and associated behavior continually create highly stressful events. The chaos that he spins, filled with temper fits that can erupt without warning (causing you Brain Freeze) are with you every day or the fear of them is.

Being stressed produces mental and emotional effects, and the often overlooked potentially deadly physical effects.

Stress damage on your body is far more serious than most people know, especially when it accrues, piles up; the damage done yesterday creates a nest for today's damage to pile on top of. The effects don't just go away, and they aren't gone just because you feel better. The real effects are lasting.

Stress produces in people (and animals) mental, emotional, and physical disturbances such as depression, anxiety, sleeplessness, confusion, forgetfulness, frustration, and more. All of those effects then become new stressors for you to cope with.

Raised blood pressure and cholesterol, damping down your immune system, digestive problems that can become deadly serious, pressure on your heart and other organs from the chemistry filling your bloodstream and fatigue, deep fatigue as your body tries to cope with the over-abundance of strong chemicals and their effects.

Most people don't understand what stress is, even though they have it and talk about it all the time. You are likely an expert at *experiencing* stress—but not likely at handling it, or stopping it.

It's impossible (and really not desirable) to cut out all stress. Stress at a healthy level gets us out of bed in the morning, sets us off to work or whatever. The goal is to keep our stress down to a healthy level. Doing that is easier when you understand what stress actually is and how it affects the body.

Most people think stress is the thing that bothers them, that upsets them—traffic jams, a boss's bad mood, a partner's snap rage. Those things are stressful, but they are not "stress."

Stress is your body's reaction to overwhelming pressure.

Stress is a physical response to mental and physical overload.

Stress is not the thing that bothers you but what you feel when bothered—pressure, agitation, unclear thinking—all the result of physical changes that occur when you encounter something bad or threatening: That's a stressor. The physical reaction is set off mentally by your brain signaling your body that you are somehow threatened, and that you need to gear up for dealing with it.

Your body's response, in preparation to survive the threat, is to instantly, at near light speed, pump out enough "upper" chemicals (made and stored in your own body) to stock a minor cartel.

Your body is wired to respond to a threat of any kind and to do so without your having to think about it. If you believe snakes are dangerous, you imprint the danger sign into your subconscious. Ever after, when you encounter a snake your rapid-fire subconscious pushes out a scream and fires up your body instantly to jump away, all before you have any rational thought.

But while you are screaming and jumping, your best friend picks up the snake and pets it. Clearly the two of you learned a different level of dangerousness for the same event—seeing a snake. Neither of you is harmed.

Fight or Flight

Say you are in your cave. Your senses pick up a threat: A scent triggers an area of your brain before you can think, or figure out what to do, "Holy Moly! I smell a saber-toothed tiger!" And Wham! Your survival chemicals flood your body. You instantly jump and run--real fast. And you can! Your survival reflexes and chemicals make that possible. You are not the tiger's lunch date.

On the other hand, if you had to parse out the various signals fro all of your senses—hearing, smell, vision, then think through the best thing to do in response, by the time you got to, "Holy Moly! It's a tiger! I'd better run!," you'd be lunch.

You see why your entire stress response system is vital to your survival.

Its major downfall is that it can get cranked up when sensing danger, fire all systems—but then there's no tiger. The result is that you're pumped up with chemistry that begins firing off nerves and muscles—but you won't go into action, so they don't get burned off. That creates a problem. Especially when, over time, it happens repeatedly. Well, when you start being alert all the time, watching out for someone getting upset and blowing up, it's as if you're continually firing up to fight or run, but you don't. Those chemicals back up; they can become toxic to your organs—and that's the damage when you don't experience catastrophe. Catastrophe fires you up too. Quite a combination.

Your response to the rush of chemicals preparing you to fight or run for your survival (even if it's only your boss's bad mood) readies you to Fight, or to run away, escape (Flight), or sometimes to Freeze (which I call mini-Bambi Brain). Freeze can be a good response if there's gunfire and you fall down; you become less a target. Not so good if there's a tiger.

All those chemicals have a job to do and they always are pumped out at the highest rate possible—because you must act instantly to survive things, much faster than you could if you had to stop and figure things out first. (The more I learn about our stress response, the more I am stand in awe of the Manufacturer. You came packaged with an automated system to enable you to survive life's dangers. And you can blame it on your body, that same response system, when you feel like throwing something, kicking something, screaming, cussing, breaking things. Handy little system, huh!

Now you know it's not because you've lost it, gone bonkers; it's just your body trying to burn off its fiery chemicals, triggered by an event you experience—or the threat of an event. Here too, the body is responding too fast for you to say, "Gee, I'm so ticked off that I think I'm going to throw that plate across the room." Thus, you can blame all such incidents on forces beyond your control.

The changes in your body that the rush of chemicals creates feel most uncomfortable. Think about it: You're jittery, jumpy, irritable, snappish. You long to do something drastic. That's the chemicals, demanding that you do something to burn them off.

> **Psych Note:** This is precisely why trying to relax when fired up never works. The only way to get relief is to get active and rapidly use them up out of your bloodstream. Walk briskly, scrub the kitchen, put on a tune and dance around, head for the gym the running course. Relaxing doesn't clear your system; then you just have to grin and bear it the pressure of wanting to throw something for hours.
>
> Our stress system was created to help us fight, not for us to fight.

Okay—if what happens to you is called "stress," what do you call the Horse's Butt (and his antics)? They are called "stress-ors."

Anything that smacks of dangerous or uncomfortable coming events is called a "stressor."

Anything presenting any kind of discomfort or threat to you, whether it does so to anyone else or not, is your "stress-or." Your stressors are yours alone. Many people take pleasure in intimidating others by crowing, saying, "Oh, that doesn't bother me at all!" If they don't say it, you get their meaning strongly of something like this: "So what's wrong with you that it bothers you?"

The traffic jam, being late for work, his attitude, snarky people, snakes. Stress-ors. And what prepares your body to deal with a stress-or? Think "the saber-toothed kind."

Right. It becomes stressed, and what you feel is called stress. Stress is really nothing more than a massive pumping of chemicals throughout your body, produced in response to what some part of your brain perceives may be harmful to you in any way. Stress produces feelings and body responses that can differ between people. (Naming stressors "stress-ers" rather than "stress-ors" would have made it easier for us, but they didn't do it that way—so we just have to make do.)

Think of stress, the physical response to a mentally sensed threat, as consisting of three areas: This will help you get a handle on it, own it, control it. Having three separate parts means there are at least three ways to approach its remedy, that you can almost always change the way you deal with stress—and the way it deals with you. Those three areas are these:

1. A conscious (and-or) subconscious memory of an experience in the past that was bad, such experience being labeled at that time as "dangerous." This is the way you are wired for survival: anything bad is instantly categorized and multiple body systems are set to go off if it approaches again, or there's even a threat of it approaching.

2. In addition, your subconscious processes, being prepared to act at light speed in the face of anything labeled "dangerous," sends masses of stimulating chemical signals all over your entire body. Your pulling back from danger is as much the result of the shock of those chemicals slamming all the nerves and muscles in your body—long before your brain has even noticed the threat (your senses notice) and in a split second you react the way you are primed to.

3. Then there's the stressor itself, and what element of it is responsible for its being classified as "dangerous."

Of those three elements of stress, which part do you think you can most easily change?

Well, the only part (besides avoiding "dangerous" events and getting specialized government training on how to hold back your reflex responses) is adjusting the degree of dangerousness your subconscious places on a given the specific threat. This can come about in several ways but usually requires a therapist. The material you generally must deal with is threatening even to think about in many cases. It doesn't take long—one session, two; the Good News is that frequently the change in how threatening something is will take place in another split-second. It will come as a flash of recognition that something that frightened you, say as a child, doesn't carry the same dangers or threat to you. When that happens, it feels like somebody just cut off the anchor that was holding you down.

Since most erroneous material in your subconscious was formed when you were a child, changing your perceptions of them is often easy. Things that were scary, or that the grownups feared (or wanted you to fear) may no longer be "dangerous" when you examine them with the eyes of today. Fear of that thing will never again have power to control you or scare you.

You can do much of this work on your own. You begin by writing about a thing you fear, like "people will "diss" me.

The Write It Out Trick

What does it make you feel like when people actually do "diss" you, then write about the way you feel when you think something is about to cause that. A few lines is usually enough for you to have a starting place on what makes you fear being "dised."

If you do have a problem in fearing the criticism or rejection of others, write a little more. Write about how and why you probably came to see that particular thing as threatening, dangerous. In the case of being dissed, for instance, you might likely about fearing that they would dislike you, drop you, and leave you outside the group. Survival depends sometimes on being inside the group, so it's no surprise that the fear of others criticism, gossip, and dissing are interpreted by your brain as a danger to you.

Step 1. Get a notebook or journal or use your keyboard; sit down and start writing. A good starter line for each of these fears you pinpoint is this:

I hate and fear criticism or mean gossip (or lies, etc.)

because it causes _____ to happen.

Step 2. Write the same kind of statement about whatever the issue in Step 1 causes to happen; in other words, I hate-fear that thing in Step 1 happening

Because it causes _____ to happen.

Step 3. Continue writing the same statement for each thing you dig up that you hate or dislike as the result of certain events until you can see you've taken it down to your automatic survival settings.

This writing exercise about what is it you hate about the "bad" thing happening can will lead you to find the heart of almost all of your fears. Use it when you feel tense; you can do this without writing eventually, just working back until you uncover what you fear that is causing your tension. Only then do you have a chance of doing the right thing to "fix" it. There's almost always underlying fear of some kind producing your tension.

You can do the write-it-out work on your own; just be sure to focus on only one thing at a time.

A session or two with a therapist who understands you are looking for short-term therapy just to work on one or two issues is a great idea if you can swing it. (Just check first whether she -- always a *she* therapist for a drinker's woman because of too many complications that block getting down to this real work) whether she agrees with one to three sessions, short-term therapy.

Short-term therapy also focuses on homework: The therapist likely will give you a raft of assessment exercises you can do at home, analyze for yourself, then bring back to her for her analysis and therapeutic suggestions.

Understanding of Your Special Kind of Stress

You and most other people focus on the stress-er, the bad behavior, the threat. We are programmed to focus on eliminating or altering a threat and that makes sense in terms of survival. At least when dealing with tigers. If he's charging, you can shoot the tiger. (Of course, you know your Inner Child will hate being in prison, so you avoid the "shooting" alternative when it's just him standing there with a drink in his hand.)

When a hot stove burns you, your mental and physical focus go to protecting yourself from further damage. You don't consider shooting the stove. You jerk your hand back. Your conscious mind decides what kind of response the specific stressor requires.

Trying to change the stressor is "Fight." What you've been doing is fighting—but his drinking is a war you cannot win by fighting it. Your strongest response is to fight the stressor, get rid of the threat, move! But you can almost never change the stress-er. You can't make the tiger lose its taste for your sweet meat. About you can do in response to a noisome stressor is Fight and Run (Flight). You can't change the tiger's preferences, nor can you change the path of a hurricane, another threat, stressor. And you cannot change an over-drinker. Which is what you have spent most of your best self trying to do.

Let's stop to evaluate where you are again: How successful has Fight (trying to change things that stress you) been working for you so far? This approach is rarely successful.

You can stop some events (the associated stressors) from occurring, like when we stop flooding by building dams, or we build hurricane-resistant homes. Or you move away from a nasty man. Those are Fight and Flight.

Fight is rarely easy (or effective), especially long-term.

Flight is, in other words, when you can't dislodge the tiger family, you consider moving the location of your hut.

You can leave town when a hurricane approaches, and move to higher ground to avoid floods. You can move out of range of a rage-aholic. These can be a form of Fight, but are more strongly based on Flight.

Flight (moving away from the stressor) is often easier than Fight, and with a misbehaving man, Flight is the only rational decision. Which is not to say it's easy, just easier than most Fight options. Flight is faster relief. And safer. Flight is almost always effective—at least in the short term. (Note the effectiveness of Move Along, which is a Flight response to your stress-er.)

On the other hand, Flight can cost you, and it's wise to consider whether you are able, or willing, to lose what it can cost. You probably have the rest of your life to come back and re-address, re-examine your decisions, as you or situations change.

You can also change the impact of a stressor by making changes to what the stressor can do to you. These attempts are Fight—building a very high fence, not keeping your cookies and honey the cave.

Again, while you can change the impact of a stress-er, it is most often impossible to change the actual stress-er. You can adjust to accommodate or avert the stressful aspects of the thing, but you will only rarely actually change the reality of the thing.

Finding new ways to react to a stressor is the very best solution.

* * *

> **Psych Note**: To see how slippery some stressors are, observe a woman who is sick and tired of the drinker's behavior, ready to separate, who may even say she hates him now, feel angry hatred.
>
> This same woman can still react at full Fight response when she finds out he's seeing another woman.
>
> A new way of seeing it is to be pleased that he may pack and go with the new love, or she can take his nastiness before he gets around you.
>
> *I Remember: There came a point for me, and for millions of other women I know, where I/we began to view his finding another woman as the greatest blessing. Yes, you may feel hurt somewhere in your little girl, but remember that what you are feeling sad about is for something you don't have anyway: his love. Now it's possible he'll go and you can begin to rebuild—again, perhaps even get a life!*

Some Fascinating Findings on Stress

Let's look at some findings from the early research on stress—back in the 1930s and 1940s. One of the first stress researchers, Hans Selye, was studying what stress was and how it affects people. In one of his first experiments, he taught rats that certain signals preceded something bad happening to them. They might be sprayed with cold water, or have a slight electric shock to their feet from the cage (such things were done early in psychological research).

Next, researchers began interrupting their little rat lives with the signals that were always followed by a bad experience.

The rats quickly learned what the signals meant, that something bad was coming (a threat). Their little bodies responded just as they were wired to: the rat chemistry for Fight or Flight flooded their systems and they began frantically trying to escape—but this time they couldn't.

Now their stress increased. First, their recognition of an approaching bad thing; second, realizing they couldn't fight or run.

After repeated trials, examination of the rats gave the science team a landmark finding. The stressed rats had quickly developed stomach lesions (ulcers).

As science and medicine then began to see, stress is not a trifling matter. Inflicting or exacerbating all manner of physical and mental problems, stress can actually kill.

In recent years, physicians have begun regularly exploring life stresses in their patients, especially when their medical conditions are not improving as expected. Medical professionals have seen that stress can cause health problems, make existing ones worse, and interfere with healing. Continuing research has found three major factors that determine the level of stress a person experiences upon encountering any stressor:

1. The intensity and duration of the stressor (the event);

2. How one perceives the stressor and what the stressor means to that individual; and

3. That individual's *perceived* ability to escape or avoid effects from the stressor.

Be warned: Therapy cannot stop the stressors. There are, however, two major areas of stressor therapy will help you:

1. Learning new ways to escape or avoid specific stressors; no longer will that stressor be experienced as inescapable.

2. Learning how to examine the way you are perceiving a specific stressor.

* * *

More Fascinating Findings on Stress

Seeing Selye's work, researchers flocked to study stress and its effects (usually using animals as test subjects, sometimes in ways that thinking people have protested and caused to end).

One team, working with monkeys, came up with another humongous finding, one that has never been adequately publicized: They accidentally stumbled upon this information that they had never before considered.

The researchers were examining whether stress from the responsibilities of leadership had bad health effects. This work was done back when people had just become aware that executives often had specific physical conditions—such as ulcers and heart attacks—and began connecting those to the stress of their jobs. They designed ways to stress monkeys and test the health effects. They put the monkeys into teams of an "Executive Monkey" and a "Worker Monkey," tying them together back to back and putting each team in a separate cart.

They taught all that a buzzer or flashing light signaled some bad-to-a-monkey event that would follow that signal. The "bad event" (to a monkey) would be a slight electric shock (illegal nowadays), a terrible loud noise, or a spray of cold water. They let all monkeys experience the signal and then the bad event.

Next, they taught Executive Monkeys what buttons on the dashboards in front of them could stop the bad event's coming. Finding and pressing the right button among several with fear of a bad consequence was presumed to simulate the stress of making executive decisions.

Once the monkeys were prepared, the experiment proper began. The buzzer/flash went off. Executive Monkeys began frantically searching for and pressing the correct button. For those who failed, both monkeys in the cart got the "bad event."

When the signal came, all monkeys, Workers and Executives, instantly flew into high agitation, shrieking, howling, struggling to get loose to avoid the bad thing they knew was coming.

Shrieking and struggling to get free, they were all in a state of extreme anxiety. Then, when the sharp, cold spray or light actually came, or a shock or awful noise, their howls and shrieks escalated. Executive Monkeys weren't always able to respond correctly. And all monkeys found that their best attempts to escape weren't working; all knew that after that noise they could not escape the Bad Thing to come. They knew they were powerless, unable to stop the process, escape, or avoid the Bad Thing.

(I wonder if you're feeling something in your gut right about now. Maybe the sense of escalating anxiety and being powerless, knowing something bad is going to happen? I should think so.)

In this experiment, the Executive Monkeys's ability to respond was blunted due to their anxiety, stress chemicals now pumping through their bodies and interfering with their brains and reflexes. They too were affected not only by dread of the bad thing coming, but also their recognition of their powerlessness to stop it.

Scientists no doubt were pleased to see that that the shrieks and screeches of the Worker Monkeys put extra pressure on the

Executive Monkeys, meaning they experienced still more stress.

At first, after "bad things" were delivered, the monkeys were able to settle down as things start moving normally again.

Then, suddenly, the buzzer or light would go off again and all monkeys would explode into struggling and screeching. Soon they no longer settled back down.

After completing a series of these tests, researchers began the work of determining what, if any, physical differences (mostly in their blood chemistry) would be observable and attributable to stress. They compared the levels of stress hormones of Executives and Workers.

What do you think they found?

They found that all monkeys were stressed, and that *many* developed diagnosable physical problems, stress disorders.

But that wasn't what shocked the researchers—and a mass of scientists and psychologists around the world. What shocked them was finding *that the monkeys who developed the most and worst stress disorders were not the Executive Monkeys! It was the Worker Monkeys! The ones whose welfare had rested on someone else who didn't do a good job of taking care of business.*

Now does it feel familiar?

This was probably the earliest hint the world got about how stress affects everyone, but especially those who were affected by other people's decisions and behaviors.

When an Executive Monkey (the one in control) didn't respond correctly (didn't do right), bad things happened to the Worker Monkey—the Bad being a result of his actions, not theirs, yet the worse penalty landed on them.

Worker Monkeys could not change or escape consequences brought on them by the actions of their partners. The "penalty" they suffered and could not escape was not of their own making and they were powerless to intervene or stop it. Also powerless to escape--trapped.

Outcome: The monkeys who developed the most serious health and emotional problems weren't the Executive Monkeys at all, as was the popular belief at the time. The worst affected were those who suffered consequences due to someone else's behavior but who had no power to change it.

The monkeys's experience of high stress was short-term and never repeated, but in that short time, they developed health problems.

Your stresses and similar experiences are ongoing. They aren't short-term. And your cruel treatment is still legal.

So what are you going to do to take care and protect of yourself from the worst effects of stress?

> **Psych Note**: Another team of researchers, many years ago, assigned points to various types of stressors so they would have a measure to compare stress levels in people. They comparing people's stress levels by the number of mental and physical problems each had. In so doing, they showed conclusively that an individual's physical, mental, and emotional problems increased with their stress levels. The higher the stress level, the higher were the physical, mental, and emotional health problems.

As partner to an over-drinker, you have above-average levels of stress. It is imperative that you understand the effects of stress, and learn to recognize your own signs of being stressed so you know when to back off or Move Along. Otherwise, it is only a matter of time until that stress rips away your emotional control, and worse, takes its toll on your body and your mind.

Usually it's the mind that's affected first. You forget things. You lock yourself out of the car. You find yourself driving but can't remember where you're going.

If you've had these experiences and have felt some concern over them, the Good News is that it's not likely dementia or Alzheimer's, and you're not going crazy. Such things are just more unwelcome effects of stress—and its unburned chemistry.

So . . . How Has Stress Affected You?

Let's find out. To understand the ways stress has been affecting you, especially in your day-to-day functions, read through the following list of the signs of stress. Some of these signs you may have can be from other experiences, before you ever hooked up with your guy, leftovers from previous relationships perhaps (not necessarily romantic relationships, like childhood).

If you had any of these stress signs and health problems before your current situation, they likely will become more pronounced as your stress load increases. And it's not just the amount of chemicals in your blood that's the problem; it's their accumulated effects on your body cells.

Check any of the signs of stress below that you have experienced:

_____Your thoughts often stray from the task at hand.
_____Worrying more.
_____Feeling anxious, nervous.
_____Easily distracted.
_____Often distracted.
_____Memory problems.
_____Locking yourself out of your house or car.
_____Becoming more irritable.
_____Becoming more withdrawn.
_____Frequent confusion, including confusion about your partner and your relationship.
_____Becoming more sensitive to criticism, ridicule, sarcasm.
_____Your sense of humor diminishes.
_____You rarely feel secure.
_____You frequently feel insecure.
_____Everyday functioning has become more difficult.
_____Obsessing on a memory of something someone has done or said.
_____Often, when you manage to pull yourself off unpleasant thoughts, they come back.
_____You have less self-esteem, less sense of your own worth.
_____You have less self-confidence.
_____You begin having emotional blow-outs, explosions.
_____You begin blowing up over small things.
_____You begin blowing up at people who don't deserve it.
_____You sometimes worry that you are losing your mind.
_____You have very little fun.
_____You frequently dread things—his drinking, his coming home, not coming home, things not going right, your own blowups.
_____You rarely look forward to things anymore.
_____You have trouble sleeping; thinking and worry keep your mind churning.
_____You take medication for anxiety, depression, or sleep problems.
_____You often feel sad.
_____You frequently feel trapped—and nowhere to turn.
_____Your personality seems to be shutting down.
_____You've become numb to what he does or says.

_____You find yourself just sitting, staring with a blank mind.
_____For relief, you've begun drinking too.
_____Your sexual desire is waning—or gone.
_____You feel too insecure or unattractive for a chance at a new love.
_____Your health is affected. Examples:

Digestive problems, including
_____heartburn
_____bloating
_____constipation or diarrhea
_____ulcers

Body structure problems, such as
_____ most headaches
_____ neck, shoulder, or back pain
_____ sore and pulled muscles
_____ leg cramps

Immune system effects, such as
_____ catching more colds (or flu)
_____ getting infections
_____ injuries or illnesses that don't heal as well or as fast as in the past
_____ previous health problems are worsening

Mental Health effects: Some examples:
_____ Nightmares
_____ Feeling depressed
_____ Feeling anxious
_____ Things that make you feel like you're cracking up
_____ You've thought of suicide
_____ In desperation and desolation, you too have tried suicide.

How many checkmarks have you made? _____

Using your checklist, how do you assess your stress effects?

_____

_____

I am concerned about mental and emotional damage you've likely suffered, also concerned about the physical effects. Many of you have been suffering these without realizing that it has been the stress causing or exacerbating your problems. I'm asking you to take your completed checklist to your primary care doctor and give her/him a true picture of the amount of stress you live with or have lived with. This will immensely help him-her in working with you on *any* physical or emotional problem. This is even more important if you see a specialist: from fungus to cardiovascular or any chronic illness, stress has devastating consequences.

* * *

What Does Your Checklist Suggest?
Some of you may be overwhelmed by the number of effects from stress that you now can see. That Bad News, however, will surely turn to Good News when you use that knowledge to spur on making important changes. Following is a rough interpretation of what your answers may be telling you about your stress level.

Checking one to five items is about what most women who are not with an over-drinker will score. This score suggests that your stress levels are probably about average.

Checking six to ten items signals that you are trying to handle more than you have resources for. (Remember that hardly anyone on earth would have more resources for coping, so this result is not due to anything lack in you.) Rather, this score simply informs you that too much is piling up on your wagon . . . you're getting too much air in your balloon . . . too much water is backing up behind your dam. Got the picture?

(Note: Each of the listed signs can be a warning all on its own; all are your body's way of warning you that you need to change something—to do something differently. You can start using them that way now, as notes of warning that you need to slow down and check what's going on and do what you need to do to take care of yourself. From now on, when illness or bad moods strike, look at what sort of stress you've been chugging along under. No magic wand is going to change him—or the

stress falling on you from his unchanged behavior. What **can** *be changed though is how you think about and handle the things that tend to create your stress. Or you can program in the signal to move farther away from the source of that stress. Remember that you are using up your only supply of resources—not because you're doing things wrong, but because you've been strapped into this ride that is being controlled by someone else. Someone who is steadily losing brain cells. So long as you attribute your discomfort to the true cause, you'll do fine. What destroys more of you is when you attribute your discomfort to some lack in yourself.)*

Checking eleven or more items indicates that your stress level is far too high, that you are in danger of starting to crack at your weakest points. At these levels, stress is likely already affecting your mental, physical, and emotional health. It's time to start looking for remedies. But, of course, you've already started that by picking up this book! In this case, I'd say your next step will be a physical checkup.

If you choose to stay in this relationship, you might stop now and seek out further help to start changing what may be happening inside you. Get a counselor or trusted friend to help you sort out your unique situation and work with you to find ways to change those things that can be changed. For many of you, much of it will be amenable to your attempts.

(Note: Examples of resources to begin working on these things are support-teaching group such as Alanon, getting individual counseling from a licensed therapist or a counselor at your local women's center. If your area doesn't have one of those, you might take a look at how you can help get one started. Meeting even one woman in a similar situation can be a great boost; you can likely arrange this through a doctor or a minister, even if he's not your minister, or of another denomination. Even a school counselor—they usually know it all!)

* * *

Ugly Words, Ugly Intentions

What makes his ugly words hurt so badly? It's that you believe them, *and* believe he really means them. But neither is the case. One thing for sure, his total intention in saying mean things is to *hurt* you. You probably say to yourself, "Oh, I know he doesn't really mean those things," but that's not the point. The point is that he is saying them. He likely doesn't mean them, but what would cause a person to say such mean things to another person except the desire to hurt them.

We're discussing this because it too is an example of behavior that is *not* love.

There is no love in the person who says mean things to his partner just to hurt her, to put her down, to make himself feel superior or get the upper hand. No, ma'am; none of that can occur in the case of true love.

As to taking in whatever mean thing he says about you, Well, Duh! Girl! This man, if he's reached even Middle Stage, is seriously mentally impaired!

I mean, how reliable are his opinions? Would you go into business with someone of his mentality?

So why do his comments get in so deep? Hurt so bad?

It's because of your deep desire and need for love. You are not a needy person except as a hungry person would be needy. To function you need a quota of love and respect, and when deprived of those things, you begin to crack at the seams.

Whether he means the mean things he says or not, he's missing chunks of brain. He can't even walk straight sometimes so who is he to be passing judgement on you??

You're already seeing that he just says things he knows will get the response he wants. Usually you getting really upset.

Indeed, that is one fact you can use to test him: When his words don't affect you, what does he do? He gets nastier. He's willing to get very nasty to force you to react the way he wants you too—which is a tantrum, or tears, or cussing, or whatever.

What he says about you is not about truth! Up until now, you have fallen back when he says the mean things, almost cringing, then mentally dug into yourself and found—oh! no! I'm not perfect! and then gone into "Oh, I'm an awful person" kind of self-torment.

His words are his weapons. Don't forget that.

Whether he uses a slingshot or an elephant gun, he's out to put you down enough that he can feel on top and go and do what he wants to do. He uses his words to fend you off, but also to deliberately hurt you.

You've seen that he can say something one minute, but later

he says, "Oh, you know I don't mean that!"

You know he'll probably say these words so, in your head, once he starts, tell yourself that he's mentally impaired, he has very poor judgement, he says things just to hurt you, and later he's gonna tell you "Aw, I didn't mean that."

None of these ways to avoid emotional injury, however, mean that now you should be able to put up with verbal abuse. No! Do not! You are worth more than that. You are more than that.

One tactic, though, is when he starts, to mentally hear him simply reciting the Pledge of Allegiance. How upset would you be if all you hear is "I pledge allegiance to the flag . . . ." Thinking this at the time will also keep it from sinking in like a knife. I promise you.

You can learn a lot by studying what kind of threat his various words create for you. This process can help you dig deep and make some deep life-changing adjustments. Fast.

You are becoming equipped to float right through many of your Inner Child's deepest fears. A brisk Move Along in the face of a stressor (especially from him) lets you mentally and emotionally regroup; the activity clears out the chemicals in your brain for clearer thought, the very same chemicals that depress you and pull you down.

While not a physical threat for many of you, certainly all of his "stuff" is a threat to your wellbeing—mental, emotional, and physical because of the stress it creates.

His bad behavior in most cases tears up circuits in your Manufacturer-made wiring. His behavior shakes your nest like a hurricane would. As a female (human, tiger, or warthog), you are heavily wired, like a rattlesnake or a mama bear, to react powerfully to any threat to your nest.

No, you are not going crazy!

Our discussion of stressors and the stress you live with should explain why your nerves have been shot—if they have. Your body is shot up with adrenalin much of the time; its effects slam every organ in your body. Chemical interference attacks your brain. This is why you have difficulty focusing, can be forgetful, can become so distracted, can sleep or eat too much or too little. None of that is because you have a mental disorder! It's pure stress. Nor are depression, anxiety, and mood swings signs that you are crazy. While some people classify these problems as mental disorders, you will not accept that judgement anymore. These things for you are purely the result of stress chemicals pounding you with very little let-up.

Would you diagnose the "anxiety" of the monkeys in the research story as a mental disorder? Or the "depression" of the dogs in the other in research as a mental disorder?

I hate to tell you, but this is precisely what has been happening in the field of medicine and mental health.

Of course you would not attribute the animals's symptoms to a mental disorder! And neither are your effects just symptoms of mental disorder. You are reacting the way all sane people react to specific stressors.

Depression results from a sense of being helpless in the face of a painful situation—and an overdose of anxiety, all the text books teach. Anxiety seems a natural and healthy reaction of being helpless in the face of something bad coming.

None of your symptoms are mental disorders. Like (and perhaps a form of) Post Traumatic Stress, they are the natural outcome of the stress an individual has lived through.

(On a lighter note: The only thing we've talked about that some may consider a mental disorder would be your continuing attempts to change these things using the same old tactics that have already failed you again and again, using that same old recipe with the same amount of rosemary. Doesn't make sense, does it? Recognize it for what it is—a lack of knowing anything better.)

* * *

Stress and You

Surprisingly, the most damaging kind of stress doesn't come from suffering a tornado or a house fire. The most damaging kind of stress is the stress that, even when small, occurs frequently, repeatedly, over and over.

One of the most common ongoing stressors for you likely is the ever-present fear of another explosion from him, a pop-rage—a debacle, an uproar—which will lead to loud mean words and loudly blaming you for "making him" upset.

This is such an awful experience for many of you that you feel anxiety and stay attentive, trying to prevent any upset, continually trying to avoid doing anything that upsets him. Not to please him so much as to save yourself being the brunt of his rage and nastiness. Staying on guard eternally means you are repeating the subconscious experience of one of his explosions continuously.

Hey, if you have so much power to make him do bad things—where does all that power go when you try to make him do good things? Come on! Keep that reality firmly pressed into your heart.

Our bodies seem to cope with large bursts of stress—but only when they are few and far between. Two stressors in close proximity will take more than twice as long to recover from.

The child in many of you believes what she was told so long ago, that changing whatever they complained about would be the solution—that then you would be loved, if only you lived up to those standards. When you didn't, you were told you caused all kinds of bad behavior on their part. That wasn't true either.

Many of you have come to believe that you are weak. Not! Consider that the strongest men in our country are torn down by ongoing stress. Dreading a blast coming at any moment. Always alert. Gee, this is sounding familiar too.

Living with an over-drinker can be very much like living in a war zone, especially in terms of how much stress you may be carrying. Frequent hurtful criticisms, potshots, traps, betrayals, lies, explosion, the surprise grenades, and there's always the possibility of a missile falling out of nowhere.

What happens to you when a stressor appears is what happens to all healthy people when one of their stressors appears (except for those who have been highly trained, like lawmen and therapists). Anyone who even implies that you are weak because of your stress reaction is mistaken or else they are working to keep you down and easy to control. And make themselves feel superior at the same time. You can see how rewarding putting you down can be to an ugly person.

Feel stress building? Get Active, Move Along, Thought Switch, Go Do Something Fun.

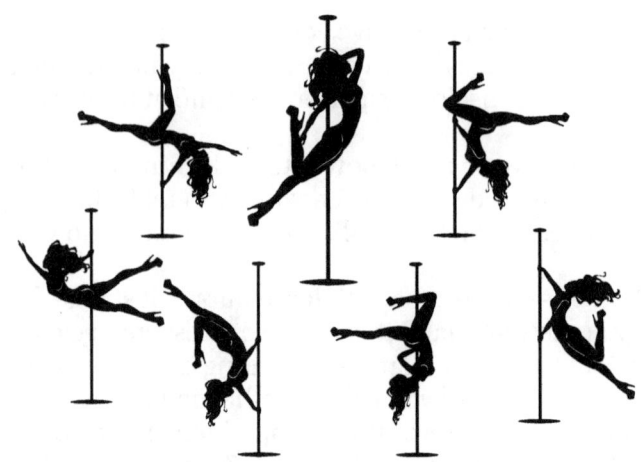

Some of the Old Remedies Won't Work for You—But Then Again, Some Will!

As you have seen, the old remedy of "Oh, just sit down and relax," after experiencing a stressor doesn't work. But the old remedy, "Get your mind off it!" turns out to be excellent advice.

But how in the world can one do that? How can one get their mind off someone shaking your nest? We're going to add a small piece to that old remedy, "Just get your mind off of it!"

1. Get active. Move Along, briskly; then Thought-Switch, to one of your dreams or goals. Now you've taken focus off the stressor temporarily. Those thoughts can burst back in, but you need only to repeat the same process. Soon it will be on auto-run

2. Replace thoughts of the scene with figuring out what's the next step toward a dream or goal.

As soon as you Thought-Switch, the chemical pumps shut down. It may take moments of activity to burn off what's already racing around your system, but the pumping stops.

Be sure to give yourself the pat on the back or butt for every tiniest bit of progress you see yourself making in every tiniest bit of what we're doing here. (Your subconscious is almost as susceptible to reward as to danger. Reward yourself—liberally, and often! If anyone deserves it, it's you.)

(Note: A caution regarding how you reward yourself. Do not reward yourself with something you already have a

problem with. Brownies or a shopping spree can feel rewarding, but only in the short term. While briefly rewarding, which is why they are so hard to kick, they can end up doing more harm than good. What was meant to be a reward ends up adding still more stress by making you feel fat and ugly.)

The Surprise Joy Trick

1. Catch it! Catch it the moment you recognize that he's "doing it again" (whatever "it" is). (You recognize it by your body: you tense up, your facial muscles, shoulder and neck tense up; you may notice you are making fists.) And once you catch it --

2. Let Your Inner Actress Rise. Put on a sweet, concerned face, and speak in a sweet tone that you don't feel.

3. Say tenderly: "Oh, you've had a rough day. Here, let me get you a beer (drink)." Then do just that. (Yes, I know you hate the drinking, BUT your Inner Actress is creating a positive scene well worth bearing with it.)
(The look on his face is the trick's first reward.)
(His falling abruptly silent may be the next reward.)

Keep in mind that surprise may block his brain briefly, so as soon as you sweetly give him the drink, Move Along. Refuse to respond to anything he says next. Act as if you didn't hear him, and keep Moving.
He may also shut down, or stammer, or pretend to refuse your offer of a drink, but once he sees the beer can or bottle or glass, another part of his brain shoves out all else.
If he protests, stay silent, Stretch 'Em, and just wait. It should take only seconds.
(Unless you're in the mood to seduce him—now, while he's still able—Stretch 'Em, Clamp 'Em, and Move Along.)

More About Your Stress Response
You've seen that The Manufacturer installed wonderful mechanisms to ensure your survival.

**Your survival mechanisms
can make you stronger and faster.
They don't, however, make you smarter!
They usually have a dumbing-down effect.**

I can't emphasize this common "dumbing-down" strongly enough! Being upset blocks your usual quick intelligence. Being aware of this glitch, however, can save you from trying to react too fast and making costly errors. Move Along is perfect for giving your own brain time to unfreeze.

When you catch yourself trying to make a decision while emotions are flowing, just hold up on the decision. Take some time. Wait until the emotion has passed to make your judgements and decisions. And remember that you can speed up the process with a brisk walk.

Another point to block negative comments making an impact: Any person's stress triggers have little to do with what stresses other people. The biggies are usually the same, but not the rest of it. No one can treat you as inferior because you are stressed by anything! And you now know that your reactions to a given stressor don't have to be the same as anyone else's either.

Increase the Power of Your New Tricks

The most effective practice of a trick is an imaginary practice where you also imagine that the stressor is present. See yourself doing each step of a trick brilliantly, successfully, and smiling proudly when he isn't looking.

How about a run at it now. Picture it: It's another night. He's at the door, a can of beer in his hand. He says something very upsetting. Flash! What do you do? How would you like this to turn out? Yes, you use the energy flooding you. Actually, your anxiety chemicals that we've established are also get-up-and-go chemicals—so you use it for your profit. Clamp 'Em! Stretch 'Em! Move Along! Now imagine your satisfied smile as you go on to do something fun.

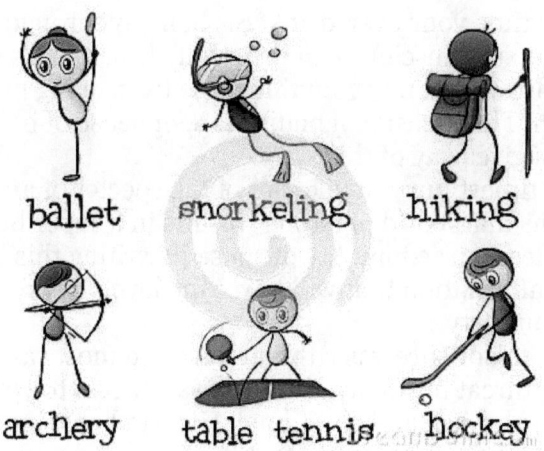

ballet snorkeling hiking

archery table tennis hockey

Until now, you've likely responded to things he says (such as "You're crazy!" or "You never do so-and-so!") as if what he said were true, or that he really believed those things. You've responded as if he was actually qualified to make judgements on your fitness! But let's stop there! Ask that beautiful little girl inside you if she will let her emotional balance depend on the words of a mentally impaired person.

What's your answer, beautiful child? _____

Looking Closer at Your Stress-ers

If you believe snakes are dangerous, you imprint the danger sign into your subconscious. Ever after, when you encounter a snake your rapid-fire subconscious pushes out a scream and fires up your body to jump and jerk away, all before you have a rational thought.

But while you are screaming and jumping, your best friend grabs the snake and starts petting it. Clearly the two of you learned a different level of dangerousness for the same event— seeing a snake. And neither of you was harmed.

Say you are in a jungle. Your senses pick up a signal of threat: "Hm-mm, I smell a saber-toothed tiger!" That scent hits your brain before you can think about it or mention it. Wham! Flight chemicals flood your body. You jump and run rapidly. You are not lunch.

If you had to think about the ramifications of that tiger smell before your feet would fly, you would be lunch.

By the time your over-drinker is halfway through the Middle Stage, your subconscious can be so full of "danger" signals that they can drown out most anything else from being processed in your brain. The occasional blank stare or sense of being in a stupor is a giveaway of this state.

Every tiniest nip you take out of the specter of any one of those items marked "dangerous" results in a super helping of mental release, freedom. My purpose in writing this book is to give you information that will lower the levels of dread I know most of you carry.

His behavior surely is a threat to you in most cases. While not a physical threat for many, certainly as a threat to your wellbeing, physical and emotional. His bad behavior signals the possibility that your nest is about to be tumped over. And you, a female, extensively wired heavily to react strongly to interference with your nest, react with the fervor of fighting for your life. Which is not crazy! It's nature, working the way the Manufacturer set it up to.

Our discussion of stressors and the stress you likely live with should let you understand why your nerves have been shot. They are shot—shot up with adrenalin, whose effects proceed to slam every organ in your body. Such chemical interference with your thinking brain is why you have difficulty focusing, get distracted, why you sleep or eat too much or too little. It's not because you have a mental disorder! Your bouts of depression and anxiety are not signs that you are mentally ill. For the most part, it's the stress chemicals—what they do to your body and brain.

Your task over the next five years or so is to begin reassessing all the things that threaten you. Most will succumb to being examined with adult eyes and understanding, and the new ways of coping you're learning.

I know that seeing how deeply you may already have been affected is a stressor in itself, but—like so many other truths in this book—if you don't learn about this and think about it, those bad effects will continue, with or without your understanding. They will do the same damage with or without your understanding. But the only way you can dump those bad effects is by understanding them and learning a few simple tricks. Stress effects aren't good, and hearing about them is Bad News, but knowing what they are how they work give you the power to change all that. And that's Good News!

Stress, very much a killer, can also cause you to get sick in a multitude of ways, then make it extremely difficult to get well.

> **Psych Note**: Research shows that apparently all human illness has a stress component. It can create health problems, or exacerbate those already existing.

Either a health problem is the direct result of stress, or stress complicates its healing. Research finds that stress even interferes with the healing of broken bones, with any kind of healing.

Most people can look back and see that many illnesses (especially colds and flu) have accompanied or followed stressful periods in their lives. Research also shows that stress depletes the immune system, so recovery from these stress-inflicted problems is also shut down. Stress can create physical harm, then depresses your immune system, making it more likely you will develop an illness; then slow prevents getting well.

Stressed people have more accidents. It interferes with paying attention. Stress warps your judgement; stress takes the edge off your abilities, talents, skills, intelligence.

Knowing these things can make you more aware and more careful during any form of stress. (It can also be a very strong motive for making some changes.)

When you are under stress, as soon as possible get active! Stay as active as you can; only activity can burn off the confounding chemistry. It won't necessarily make things better, but it will halt damage to your body from backed-up stress chemicals and it will allow you to relax, and get your brain working again. Don't try to relax! Get active.

More stress relief info

Write on your wall somewhere, "Be Gentle With Yourself!" That's a sweet way of reminding yourself to get off your own back.

From now on, it's Good News when you make a mistake! Life just gave you another opportunity to practice your new ways. Especially your new ways of treating yourself.

Mistakes aren't the end of the world, although your Inner Child is imprinted with that idea. And, of course, you're going to list that now and begin to work on that fear-stressor now.

Every, every, every-body makes mistakes, girl. Lots of 'em. Do you think you're really better than all the other humans in the world? So much better that you won't or shouldn't make mistakes? Who convinced you of that? Avoid such people where possible, and keep your contacts brief. This allows you to become strong without intermittent attacks of criticism or looks of silent scorn.

And who might such "someones" be?

_____

_____

_____

Right now! Stop the harsh judgements on yourself! When you catch yourself at it, apologize to that Beautiful Inner Child and tell her how precious and good she is. No one can do that for you.

And it's amazing how fast this trick will start making a difference. (That's your subconscious again, working for you) It really feels good to get off your own back, and your little piggie subconscious gobbles up all that good feeling and prods you on to "do it again!"

Who's Not Sleeping?

You have likely learned that lack of sleep is itself an extreme stressor. Lack of sleep means your body and mind are not getting the required time to recharge itself. You are like a cell phone that needs to plug in nightly for recharge.

Your brain keeps tabs on all your body processes, all the time; it knows (subconsciously) better than you (consciously) know what your energy-mental-emotional level is at any given moment. Other parts of your brain rely on getting that information, especially in the split seconds when you meet a stressor

Your subconscious keeps tabs on how "up to it" you are in the face of a stressor. When you are sleep-deprived, it's an additional stressor working on you. Lack of sleep slows all your processes, makes you far more likely to make bad decisions, mistakes. These, in turn, produce still more stress, further reducing coping abilities.

Some of the things you may be doing now thinking they are in your best interest—such as trying to solve a problem anywhere near bedtime—set you up for failures the next day. These problems like to pose as something you must do now for your survival; in reality, doing it in the evening will rob you of tomorrow's strength.

Another example of habits that may be tearing you down is arguing with him: First off, because it's useless! You now know that you cannot win an argument with him—and have it stick. Secondly, he just becomes more irate and you become more frustrated—with the accompanying juiced-up stress chemistry peaking in the stay-awake mode.

You've nothing to lose with your "Yes, Honey Trick," if you can throw out a little bull yourself should he press you. Your Inner Actress will love it! Let her out to play.

His Sleep Loss vs. Yours

Over-drinkers complain a lot about not sleeping well—about being tired all the time. They blame the mattress, the noise, the kids, the neighbors, you.

But their sleep loss, though detrimental, is quite different from yours: The drinker loses sleep because of what the alcohol is doing to his body and brain (which, note, is accomplished while doing what he considers having fun—and actually is a brief escape from stress for him).

Your sleep loss happens because of worry, anger, fear, and hurt. Stress now robs you of sleep. You are utterly miserable. He's having what he thinks of as fun. You're miserable.

What do you plan to do about that?

What's more, their "sleep" isn't real sleep. It's more "passing out," which is an entirely different brain state from sleep. Passing out is a near-comatose level of brain function. There's no Rapid-Eye-Movement (REM) (the phase of sleep where you have eye movement under sleeping eyelids).

REM is the all-important, deep, restorative, immune-recharging sleep. He's not getting it. He's not being restored, recharged. He's being poisoned, his body damaged—no wonder he's always tired.

> **Psych Note**: The major reason over-drinkers complain of being tired all the time is because they are dosing themselves with a toxic drug, at higher than toxic levels.
>
> They are actually poisoning their bodies. No wonder they feel tired and run-down. They are killing their bodies.

Another huge difference between the drinker's loss of sleep and yours is that when a problem drinker has trouble sleeping, he simply ups his dose of "medicine" (a drink or other substance--including prescription drugs).

Many of you have begun searching for sleep aids, but found they make you feel dull the next day, which means your attempt to lower your stress has created another stressor. Take great care with sleep aids; be sure you and your doctor consider your greater-than-usual need for coping energy when discussing them. He may not realize your stress load or your need for a clear head. Tell him about your mate's over-drinking. (Unless he is also an over-drinker, he will understand and work with you for the best choice.) Choose the sleep aid with the least bad effect on you, and you'll have to experiment to find one.

Recorded relaxation exercises also help many drinkers's women sleep. I too have used them. They are a wonderful way to turn your mind away from things you can't solve during the day. Unlike reading, listening doesn't stop when you get distracted by another thought—the information keeps flowing in at some level.

In fact, I heartily recommend that you try the healthy teas known to aid in relaxing and sleeping, along with recorded relaxation guides, and prayer or meditation—all before going for another sleep medication. Anything you can do naturally is definitely worth a little more effort; that's because most medications have unwanted side effects.

As you lie down at night, deliberately turn your mind to searching for one good thing that happened in your day, and one good thing you accomplishes. (Because a positive answer is important, if all else escapes you, remember that your hair didn't fall out!) This thought, along with a sense of gratitude for that or something else that went right today, are the most effective relaxers at bedtime. They can shove aside worry, obsession, plotting. Tomorrow is soon enough to get back to that.

(Note: In later stages of deterioration, a drinker may be unable to stay asleep for more than a few hours at a time. You

may not be as aware of this if you have learned to sleep through his thrashings, or if you now sleep elsewhere—due to his noise, his smell, or his peeing the bed.)

Sex is a great relaxer

Sex with an over-drinker may not be great—but sometimes it's better than none. (Offer to get him Viagra if needed. Erectile dysfunction arises quite early in over-drinkers, as early as their 20s for those who started drinking when younger.)

Or just get him another beer and give it a go at getting him in the mood. You're not going to stop the drinking, so let's begin to use it to your advantage occasionally.

I bring this up to remind you that most bodies need regular, satisfying sex. Being held. Being wanted. Being hot! Orgasm. These are extremely important elements of life for humans. And you are human. You may have tamped down your feelings for so long, that seems unattainable, but rest assured—with a lover who knows the tricks and also knows a woman's needs, you'll soon agree it's one of the best things in life. The intimacy. The caring.

Of course, if the caring isn't there, it rarely is satisfying to women. To men, yes—but only rarely for women.

Bring out your Shameless Inner Actress frequently and hand everything over to her. She can handle it from there. (You know what you like, so let her pretend to be a school teacher to a bad boy, giving him "special" instructions. He'll love it!)

(I won't advise you further regarding sex here, because it is an individual experience. Each of us has her own sense of "rules." On the other hand, let me point out that many of your "rules" aren't your own.) Discuss sex with friends, and-or see a counselor to do this. One session should be sufficient to get a new perspective on your sexuality. Living with an over-drinker can have terrible effects on one of your greatest stress releasers!

Check it out: You may be robbing yourself of a lot of joy and fun without knowing it. For sure, most bodies function at their peak when sexually satisfied.) Go on-line and research books on sex; buy them or try to find them at your local library too; you may be surprised at how some libraries have loosened their strict rules. New sex books are usually best. There's so much information out there nowadays and writers are so comfortable with the topic. Many of the older books were guarded, even implied that sex was bad. Newer books are open in discussing sex and finally make room for individual differences.

More Stress Research

Decades ago, researchers discovered a condition that looks like depression, tests like depression—but it isn't true depression. They aptly named it Learned Helplessness. This form of depression arises, not so much because of bad events, but because of one's inability to escape those bad events.

It appears to be part of human (and animal) wiring to give up at the point one realizes her-his efforts are not successful, realizing that nothing she knows is helping, and she's wearing down. When she wears down, she has a deeply held belief that nothing else can help.

Of course, when you're not caught up in it, you can see that isn't true; it comes because your subconscious believes that if it doesn't know another way, there must not be one. At that time, there's a giving up. No more searching for solutions, no more feeling much of anything. This is likely a survival option.

* * *

Researchers were testing animal responses to stress when an experiment (using dogs and cats), set up an inescapable "bad thing." An inescapable bad event.

They placed dogs in separate cages wired to deliver shocks to the bottoms of the dogs's paws (illegal today). They were trying to stress the animals enough to make them try to escape, after researchers had made it impossible for them to escape by wiring closed all the cage doors.

Most of these experiments had no warning signal, so the animals never knew when the shock was coming. In tests where there were warning signals, the animals would always frantically try to escape. At first.

Here's what they found: Early on, animals make energetic attempts to escape the bad conditions, attempts that always failed. After varying lengths of time, they all finally gave up, lying down in their cages. In giving up, they would lay down, right onto the electrified and shocking floor of their cages.

Once they lay down, they appeared to ignore the shocks. They ceased to react at all, even when the power of the shocks was turned up to a very painful level. This is the point where they diagnosed Learned Helplessness. The animals had learned that none of their efforts worked, and resigned themselves to their suffering. I'm glad this sort of research is no longer allowed; nevertheless, this one brought valuable research findings to help a drinker's woman understand her predicament.

Perhaps the worst part: Once the animals lay down, stopped reacting, nothing was ever able to get them going again.

The cage door could be opened and stay open, but they would not attempt to leave. They could even pick the animals up and move them out of the cages, but then the animals, rather than enjoy their freedom, stayed in the Learned Helplessness state— laying down despite other stimuli or urging.

The animals learned something: They "learned," after an extended time filled with their best attempts to change their condition, that those best efforts didn't bring the needed results.

They learned that they were helpless in the face of a bad thing. Their response was to close down, shut it all out, including the pain. They became sluggish, , nonresponsive. (In humans, these are the signs used to diagnose severe depression.)

Some of you have been diagnosed as depressed—which you probably are—but your form of depression is different from the common mental health disorder. It isn't a mental problem! It's a normal reaction to a very real and terrible situation; it occurs when one's best efforts don't get them the needed relief. Many cases of depression that don't respond to medication aren't true depression, but human cases of Learned Helplessness. It looks like depression, but it isn't quite the same. It is depression-plus. Medication for depression doesn't cure Learned Helplessness. Knowledgeable and caring client-respectful therapy bring you back to appreciating yourself and caring for the girl inside you, the True Princess.

Do not allow anyone to prescribe anti-anxiety or anti-depression medications in the belief they will solve the problem. Those only come anywhere near solving the problem when they are prescribed for him. You can refer a professional to this book and they can do their research. Most important though is for you to understand the problem and that, while you may suffer from anxiety and-or depression, and medication can ease those problems, they cannot fix it. Bringing your car in out of the tornado may shelter it, but it won't fix the damage already done.

Treating you with medication is like treating someone for poison ivy and sending her right back into the poison ivy patch.

There *are* effective therapies that can bring you back to life, to more fully experiencing the wonderful life you are capable of building for yourself. Believe me, you can become the person you were meant to be, who you really are.

Believing you've done all you can and nothing works and nothing more can be done leads to living in conditions that may require you to medicate yourself to survive. And this is no way to live. Researchers call this condition Learned Helplessness. It's what we see in women stuck in bad marriages, in relationships with nasty drunks, and physically or otherwise abusive mates. They have learned that nothing they have ever done or tried has changed their bad situation. When they truly don't have anymore what it takes to break free, they have learned that they are helpless.

These women have worked and struggled, usually for years, trying to change their conditions—without success. They have tried every method they know to avoid or escape their bad conditions. To no avail. They have run out of tricks, run out of energy, and run out of hope that it can ever get better. Learned Helplessness

They have learned that they do not have the power to change or escape their intolerable conditions.

Now we know that while animals do not appear able to escape Learned Helplessness, people definitely can. The solutions are rather simple, but many aren't easy. For example, leaving an abusive relationship is a simple statement, but not a simple act. Still, it can be done, often much easier than some believe, especially with a little help—often the best being found at a local women's shelter. Not so much for the shelter part—which is good—but for the quality of the experienced counselors. The women you will be talking to are almost all survivors of abuse themselves and can tell you what worked for them and help you learn whatever you need to.

Best of all, none of them would ever think something is wrong with you because you got into this situation! They all know how easy it to happen—and usually only to a very special kind of woman, the best kind of women. (Perhaps one day you will be the messenger to some other woman on down the road.)

Stress Relief 101

The keys to relieving stress are understanding it—and then becoming aware of your own responses to it.

Blowing up under pressure is a legitimate option for handling stress. It's a natural process, in keeping with the laws of nature, the over-stretched balloon, for example. In some cases, blowing up can be helpful—and it can feel mighty good. For a while.

But it only feels good so long as you remember how normal it is! If you start to think (or others suggest) that an emotional blowup is a sign of mental disorder, both of you are wrong. A balloon that slips out of your fingers because of all the built-up pressure, blowing all its air out in a Whooosh! is actually saving itself from being destroyed. One more puff and it might have been.

Think of stress effects like gas: it's best to let it out when it starts building up.

No! Relaxing Won't Work!

Multitudes of people, men and women, have been disappointed in themselves, feeling like failures when they can't calm their emotions with relaxation and meditation. Maybe some people (at guru level, like the Dali Lama) can. But gurus ain't us.

Perhaps, down the road, you'll get there, but at this point, you cannot quickly calm an inner storm by relaxing. Only by getting active. Fast results demand movement. The faster you Move Along, the faster your brain and body settle down and feel better.

Here's a thought: Every time he's ugly from now on, he is giving you another *exciting* opportunity to practice your new skills of Stretchy-Lip Smile and Move Along, and going to do something fun.

With all the opportunities to practice that he'll likely create, you're going to be a star at this in no time!

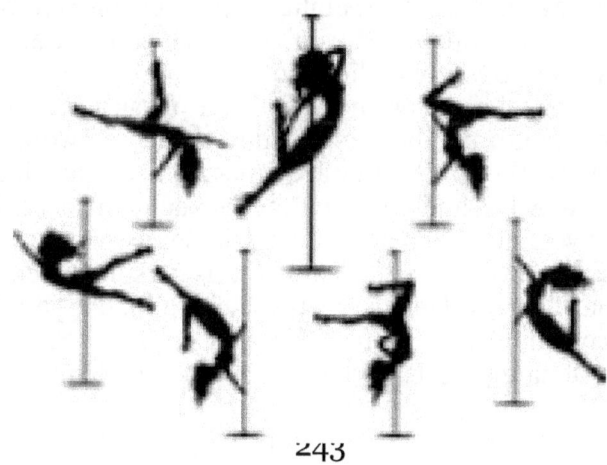

Talk About Holding Things In!
Being really good at holding in emotions isn't rewarded!
It's punished.

Holding in your emotions results in bigger blow-ups, bigger crack-ups. The better you hold things in, the bigger your eventual explosion will be. Take that to the bank!

Your solution? Learning a new trick: how to recognize and handle your stress; learning many ways to choose from at any given time. (Books and maybe short-term counseling are both extremely successful in this area.)

Those Uncomfortable Signs of Stress Can Become Your Best Friends!
Your signs of stress are your Go! button for grabbing one of the remedies that usually work for you and getting with it.

Remember that list of the signs of your stress near the start of this chapter? Now all of that which may have been scary can be turned on its head. Now you are going to use those very same signs as signals to immediately commence with a stress-relief trick. What once was Bad, now becomes Good.

Saving yourself requires gradually building the habit of keeping tabs on your stress level and you're going to do that by becoming extremely aware of every sign you usually exhibit that you are now learning are simply signs of stress. (First ask yourself if you are pushing yourself too hard. If yes, Stop it!)

The emotional blow-ups you have feared marked going nuts don't just pop out of the sky. They build up before blowing up.

You now improve your ability to protect yourself, bearing in mind that if you don't, you won't be much good for anything anyway. They'd lose you then too.

Keeping tabs on your hour-by-hour physical and mental welfare seems quite daunting to most drinkers's women. Some of it is because they know they are expected to be carrying the world, like Atlas, and have no time for such nonsense, but also because you have some to not like yourself very much. In part you don't want to be bothered with this person you don't like, in part your Learned Helplessness is kicking in. But you can do this.

Using all the signs you checked on the Stress Signs Check List isn't at all daunting. It feels good. I think it's because your subconscious grasps you're onto something really good.

If you take to heart that your emotional blow-ups and crashes always, *always* occur due to accumulated, unspent stress, and if you impress yourself with the concept—perhaps noted on sticky notes?—you will in short order become perceptive and able to use the best trick for the moment.

Something as simple as taking a short walk at about the same time every day, or working out around the same time every day, or any physical exercise—especially late in the day—has the potential of burning off all the accumulated garbage and the stress chemicals that coping with it have set rushing around your body. Your reward? No more crashes or blow-ups, better sleep, and feeling a whole lot better. The physical action combined with the mental work will leave you feeling really good. (That's why your subconscious is going to help you learn this really fast.)

> **Psych Note:** Doing something at about the same time every day speeds up forming the habit.

Not everyone stores their tension in the same way, or in the same places in their bodies. You now know where you store yours from your list of body parts affected by stress. Spend some time thinking about things that happen to you, physically and mentally, as you become stressed. Do you clamp your jaw, scrunch your shoulders, make fists, get sweaty hands, develop digestive troubles, stiff neck? Get antsy? Get irritable? All the above?

Taking time to think about this creates a giant leap toward avoiding emotional meltdowns.

So list here three to five things you're aware happen in your body—and mind—as stress begins to build.

1. _____

2. _____

3. _____

4. _____

5. _____

The Creating Comfort Trick

1. When you become aware of one of your signs of stress—Stop! Right then.

2. Take a break! Do something that works to break your stress.

3. Figure out a more useful or fun way to move toward your today-solution.

Another tip: Get in the habit of working on only one of your problems at a time. The attempt to deal with and resolve several issues at a time will do you in. The pull of your attention toward a problem is natural; what you missed (that some lucky girls got) was another trick. This part of the stress trick bag is one of the very few that are mental.

The One Rare Mental Trick Trick

1. If it's not a life-or-death issue pulling your attention from what you're doing, temporarily put this interfering issue on your mental closet shelf, in a spot where you can easily reach it and bring it back down. Stick a mental note on the mental package about a preferred time to come back and work with it.

2. If something interrupts you and bothers you, create a To-Do List and write this thing on it. You must write these things down, else they will keep running around in your head, distracting you from doing your best, and creating their own stress.

3. Once you've added that issue to your To-Do list, return your focus to whatever you were working on when this new one interrupted you and give it your full, less stressed attention.

When several problems come on you at once, take a moment to assess. You can save hours by taking these few seconds to scan the issues and select the most urgent (urgent means like the house is on fire), and deal with that single issue until it's resolved or you realize that it can't be done quickly.

Catch yourself every time you slip on your Super Girl suit.

As to stress relievers beyond getting active, you've come across many lists of these in books, magazines, pamphlets at your doctor's office, on television, and from many other sources.

I'm going to repeat some of them in a list here because I want you to have the list at hand as much as possible—until all the techniques become second nature—and they will.

Yes, it seems like a lot of work, bother, but here's the facts, ma'am: No one else is going to do any of this for you.

That doesn't seem entirely fair, since someone else put much of it on you—still, that's the way life is set up.

Absorbing that, I want you to pick no more than two items you think will be fairly easy for you to begin working on from the list below. Your goal is to gradually make that a comfortable habit, a new way that—through practice—becomes reflex, as natural as less successful tactics are now. They got that way, you recall, by practice, repetition.

You know, those lucky girls learned young that when you fall, all you have to do is brush off and get back up and keep going. Wow. What a concept. We thought you needed to stop and beat yourself up horribly. The Lucky Girls got it; now it's your turn learn these things too. (Learning doesn't generally occur if you see or do something once.)

Make a chart or use a checkmark or gold star on your calendar to show days you've done a new trick. Make no comment on days when you didn't. Of course you can't do it every day! That would be perfect, and perfect ain't us either. (I like gold stars.)

**!!VERY IMPORTANT!! Acknowledge even your tiniest successes and Celebrate them!
Every time.**

Using science to help you achieve your goals, then your dreams, make some very special mark to symbolize each time you do the new thing, or do it slightly better. Mark it like you would mark a child's growth on the wall.

Praise yourself. I still pat myself on the butt and say, "Good Girl!" when I do something good. It feels really good. What you do in that act is make real and memorable a dose of praise that can cancel one putdown, or a batch of them. Acknowledge your growth, your positive change—no matter how small you may think it is. Become a loving, praising mother to the beautiful little girl inside you, your Inner Child.

The trick is to focus on the days you're accruing with lovely marks to show your progress and achievement.

I'm going to list a few important elements of stress reduction, which are actually reducing stress effects. If you see any on the list that you'd like to try, do so, but it's best to not pull out more than one or two at a time. Start plugging them in to your schedule—on a very tiny scale—baby steps.

Working on more than two at a time is how those of us who think we need to be over-achievers shoot themselves in all five toes.

You guarantee your failure when you seek success in a flash.
What comes in a flash is sure to crash;
What comes gradually usually lasts

> **Psych Note:** Each stress-reliever you add to your repertoire makes you stronger; it also makes picking up the next one easier. So pick one or two; red checkmark them. Write them on 3x5 cards or sticky notes and post them around. If the ones you choose don't go easily, pick others. Do that as often as it takes to get a couple of them under your belt. Then confidence takes over.

SOME STRESS RELIEF METHODS

- Get adequate sleep. Changing sleep habits is a gradual process.
- Eat properly, going easy on the sugar and caffeine.
- Exercise—especially walks in lovely places. Often.
- Exercise regularly, set up a routine. Routine anchors you.
- Learn yoga or tai chi or some other form of active relaxation.
- Get CDs of relaxation exercises.
- Take long, pleasant baths.
- Do at least one thing you enjoy every day; three is better, but one is the minimum.
- Begin a program of slow weight loss if you are overweight—slow, say one pound a month. Do not allow weight loss to become another stressor.
- Sing, loudly—even if you're off key. If you think you sound awful, then sing when you're alone (and we've already established that a drinker's woman has substantial alone time).
- Laugh often, at least once every day and often at yourself.
- Get five to fifteen minutes of direct sunshine daily.
- Avoid contentious, critical, or difficult people. Just stay away

from them, or limit the time you must spend with them.
- Never waste yourself just to argue with a contentious, critical, difficult person. They will never be swayed by argument! Just make your excuses and Move Along.
- Avoid arguments of all kinds. (Be agreeable, then go ahead and do what's best for you.)
- Build your assertiveness skills.
- (Just reading over this list brings a soft stress relief!)

The slightest progress on even one of these stress-relievers, and others you find, quickly bring noticeable change in several areas of your life. In fact, stress relief techniques come as close as anything else in life to being a flash cure, immediate relief.

> The best medication for a drinker's woman
> probably is giving it to her partner.

* * *

MASTERY

Pull out one or two points from this chapter that you want to absorb totally or fast, and write them here.

1. _____

_____

2. _____

_____

Chapter 8

Making a New Plan— How to Care for a Princess

Over-drinkers wear away their woman's spirit. Every time he makes a negative comment, criticizes her, calls her names, a part of her absorbs it, and a piece of the sweetest parts of her pulls back and tucks in. And even as she argues, protests, she still absorbs it. The result is becoming more isolated because feeling inadequate, inferior, and the result of isolation is loneliness. Deep loneliness.

She's trapped into this by being human; Saints Are Not Us. She can always find something about herself and what she does. Yet it's only human. Somewhere, even before this relationship, she has picked up the idea that she must do things perfectly, be and look perfect, or suffer painful consequences (and we often suffer worse from emotional and mental pain than physical pain).

When a drinker's woman demands perfection of herself, and fails to meet it, she feels especially unworthy, and if she can dig up even a hint that there's some truth in it, she shrivels.

How do the lucky girls handle this?

They check themselves for whatever was criticized, without fear and trembling. If they find anything that matches up to the criticism, they admit it first to themselves (and the other if that's in her best interest). She may or may not assess it to be worth trying to change, or trying to change at present, and perhaps makes a note to look into later to determine if she can do anything about it, and if so, she does it. If not, she writes all of that on her subconscious for later reference, should that or a similar criticism arise again. Then drops the issue.

Not the drinker's woman. She beats herself with the imperfection, and does so regularly and likely for the rest of her life.

She doesn't easily accept that it's okay for her to be imperfect. She becomes stone when anyone talks about being human. Part of her believes it, for other people, but it doesn't apply to her. Unskilled in assertiveness, and deeply needing love, her self-defense system has no substance. Because of this, she can appear weak and she is weak—in self-protection and self-defense skills. We know she is exceptionally strong in countless ways, but not in caring for herself.

She believes that an imperfection makes her weak, makes her unacceptable. Not just any old imperfection but being imperfect in some area another person demands it from her. By the time such a woman finishes this chapter, that belief will shrivel.

We've repeated several times how powerful repetition is to imprint new ideas, strongly and rapidly. And now you realize that repetition of negative comments works exactly the same way. Repetition of negative judgements imprint the negative ideas. Through repetition of a negative judgement, you will come to believe it's true, and only repetition of the truth will sway you from that.

Every time someone else finds you lacking and shows it, or says it, that's another repetition and a reinforcement of the negative idea. When you judge yourself as lacking and think a negative thing about yourself, that's another repetition of the accusation the judgement. Certainly you lack reaching perfection! Other than that, you're just the same as every other person on the planet. Not worse. None of us have enough of any quality to be perfect; we're all struggling somewhere below that line. People around you have, in error and perhaps believing they are correct, pointed out where you fall short of perfection often enough that you now do it to yourself. Repetition of that judgement piled on the last repetition.

You lack even the basics for some self-protection. You have been shaped by others, likely from infancy, to have little care for your own welfare or needs, and to focus on pleasing or taking care of others. A foundation for a self-centered guy to build on was already there before he met her, before he began to pile it on.

Pay attention here: This quality, being more focused on caring for others probably was one of your qualities that attracted him in the first place. You believed you should show a future partner how caring you are, but the wrong kind of partner will admire it for the wrong reasons.

Some of the things he says are similar to things her parents or others said, which assures us that you have said these same things or something very like them to yourself: Repetition. It won't wishing, or "making up your mind to change" that effectively begins to change your own harsh judgements of yourself. Only correcting yourself when you do it.

Your self-concept won't respond to wanting change; change will come only as you begin applying the tricks that cause thinking to change. One of those , the Steer Your Thinking Trick, with its

Steer Your Thinking About Yourself Trick

(Note: You're getting good at working on these tricks by now, so you can handle one with a few more steps—especially since it's addressing something that goes very deep, and has likely been reinforced countless times since childhood, perhaps since infancy.)

1. **Catch It**

2. **Recognize** you are beating a wounded child—or puppy.

3. **Visualize** the wounded one and love on her.

4. **Correct your negative statement** with the Thought-Switch technique: Think of a time when you were the opposite of what you are now accusing yourself of.

5. **Focus on this memory**, proof that you simply aren't totally the negative thing.

6. **Congratulate yourself** for catching it. "You've done very well, Sweetie!"

7. **Picture yourself** while in one of your good qualities.

8. **Pat yourself on the butt** and say, "Good Girl!"

It's no wonder that a part of you so easily believes some of the awful things he says about you. Most of you have heard them before, or something similar.

* * *

> **Psych Note:** The brain only lets in what others say if you think their opinion of you is *important*.
>
> They were important to you back then, and he is important in your life now. Just because you don't like him doesn't mean he's unimportant. He may be even more important in the sense that you want to please him to avoid trouble. We are wired to pay attention to what important people say; that's how we learn all the things we need to learn. What if, around age 12, you were riding in the back seat of the family car when a teenager in a passing car shot you a bird and yelled out "You're stupid!" It would surprise you, perhaps hurt a little, but you wouldn't take it in like a sponge—the way you are wired to do with important people. By age 12 you'd know that this kid and his opinions are not very important at all so his comment bounces off an automatic, subconscious mental screen at light-speed , or a little slower if he was cute.

If a parent or teacher hollered, "You're stupid!" and their opinion of you was important to you, the label would get all the way in. So you could pinpoint it and eliminate it.

Problem is that you never learned the ways that is done.

(Note: The process of taking it in is a primary mechanism, and you became so adept with it that probably set you up to become a drinker's woman. According to how young the mean and critical things started being said to you, you may never have had a protective shield at all. You just took it all in and tried to do whatever possible to change whatever was being criticized—usually without question.)

Now you are going to begin to question any and every thing negative anyone—anyone—says to you. You will soon have the skill to bounce it off as well as the lucky girls who were taught all the good stuff and helped as she mastered it.

(Note about the Previous Note: Holding a grudge over these experiences poison you, not those who do you wrong. Worse, getting into blame blocks your ability to learn a new way to avoid getting the same treatment in the future.)

And here's another point: Even if a criticism is true, it doesn't make you despicable and unlovable.

When anyone treats you as if you are despicable or unlovable, they're off their rocker. Ask yourself each time how really important is their "opinion." While it may have been very important to that little girl we were, it really isn't to the grown woman. And it's suspect—especially when you seem to need someone who thinks so poorly of you. No matter how they claim to love you, their behavior and criticisms speak louder.

* * *

Now it's time to add more tricks to your accumulating supply.

Your learning to obsess on anything negative that others say is a flaw in you, especially when you couple it with a tendency to dismiss praise (and accepting praise is a healthy way of keeping balance). This response was part of your original wiring, but for various reasons, pleasing others and gaining love, approval, acceptance became more important to you, not because you went wrong there, but because you were building self-protective skills the only way you were born knowing how. It goes something like this: Getting upset (stirring up adrenalin that assists things to stick in memory), then focusing on what was said, then charging head-first into correcting any flaw that others accuse you of.

Your desire for and need for love is perfectly normal. It's wired in. Even animals have the need for companionship. It's a wired-in need—to be accepted, approved of, cared about, loved. Your early wiring cause you to pay attention to authority figures and model yourself as instructed. If we didn't have that, babies would never learn to laugh, talk, walk, and so on.

The process breaks down due to others's mistaken (rarely deliberately destructive) responses and teachings.

Because humans need each other to survive, being part of a group, others have to like you. Thus you learned to obsess on anything negative others said about you, to work at changing it so you would still be included, accepted.

You were given to believe that if you fixed the flaw that person pointed out, they would be very happy with you, accept you, like you, include you.

Maybe love you.

Your perfectly normal need to be loved is what causes you to focus—no, obsess—on negative things others say about you. (Always remember when you find yourself obsessing that seeking to earn love is where you learned it. You were just trying to earn love by becoming others wanted of you.)

Do you love your child when she's done something you don't like? Of course you do. You may not like their behavior at the moment, but that thing we call love, a bonding of spirits, remains.

(Think how the smart child you were to figure out a way to get the love she needed.)

We know you learned to seek love this way when you were very, very young. We know that because it had to have happened before you learned to doubt authorities.

You probably were highly accomplished at this before age 4. And likely before age 3. Wow.

How does that make you feel about yourself?

The cure? Simple, but not always easy.

- Every time your catch yourself obsessing over some negative comment someone has made, force a Thought Switch and deliberately bring to mind one of your really good qualities. (This is like slamming a positive charge onto the negative one; it obliterates the negative!)

- Now, call to mind *three* of your wonderful qualities.

- Attend to reality: You are very much a worthwhile person, that just because someone says something negative doesn't make it real—or you any less a Princess. Who ever said you were perfect and would live up to the expectations of everyone on the planet? Their negative opinion doesn't mean there's something wrong with you!

The only cure I've found for the battered self-concept is piling on "Atta boy" praise—I mean "Atta girl." At every good thing you notice doing. Begin, for at least one week, daily reciting your list of positive qualities. The inner you will respond, almost immediately, to this self-therapy. You are on your way to becoming your own best friend—and loving it.

Even animal babies are fixated on doing what the parent instructs. (Most of the time.) This wiring is to insure our survival! We enter a world we know nothing about, a world that can be extremely dangerous. Survival trumps everything, so this wiring can remain strong throughout life. As people mature and their intelligence develops, something special happens for lucky girls.

- They are taught to examine, weigh out criticism, precisely how to do that. They can observe their parents doing it.
- They are taught how to dispose of unworthy ideas.
- If a criticism is found to have merit, the lucky girls are taught how to fix the problem; they begin replacing the undesired behavior gradually with another one more suitable.

The Bad News: If your basic needs to belong, to be valued and liked, to be cared for weren't met adequately when you were young—for whatever reason, the wiring for all those things was never installed.

The Good News: All of these things can be taught—to anyone at any age.

The lucky girls were taught that negative judgements, comments, and opinions of others aren't to be absorbed like Holy Scripture. While some of us still cringe at comments from the same old negative people, and only because we've never been taught how to do these things!

You are now in the process of learning all of these things that will bring wonderful changes into your life.

One thing is to step back and reconsider: How important are those people's opinions to you today? You may need help to do this and a good counselor is a good investment in this entire endeavor.

For some of these people, you really don't care any more if they don't like you as you are. You may wish they did, but your welfare does not rest on it.

Whenever you find yourself believing that you must be perfect in order to be loved, check to see if the opinion is life-altering, if it is necessary to your survival for them to love you. If so, work with them to discover how to be more like what they want. But if they are not extremely important to your survival, set the issue aside and continue to be your wonderful self.

And go do something fun!

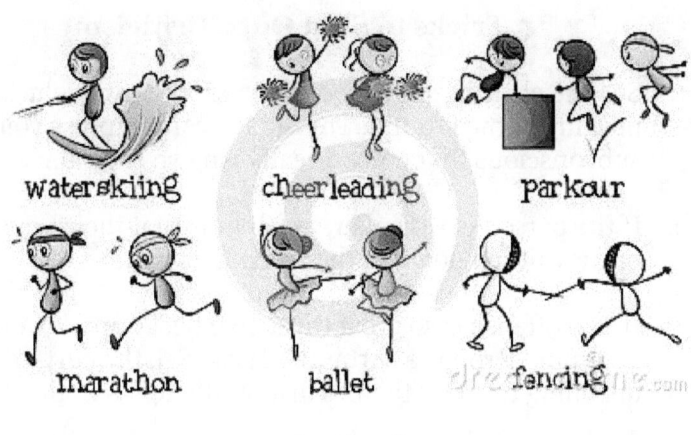

* * *

Self-Protective Tricks

Most drinkers's women have a wounded Inner Child. She needs this segment read to her, out loud, frequently—at least until you notice she's not hurting as bad as before when people are ugly or say ugly things.

I learned this trick from a great teacher; it's a "blessing" to say over such people:

> I love you,
> I bless you,
> I set you free!

"I love you." (As God loves, just because they are also spiritual beings, and when I can't say that, I only need to refrain from hating. This has worked magnificently for me—and others.

"I bless you." (I wish for you a better and happier life so you might become less critical and more loving.)

"I set you free!" And this is the part that has done the job for me. The tendency to hang on to old hurts is universal, and probably good for survival, but it has a high cost. I think I've already quoted the Dalai Lama here but it bears repeating: Hate is a poison that kills the hater.

Another great trick when you catch yourself obsessing on a person who has said something ugly is this:

3 Tricks to Shut Out a Criticism

1. See the critic hopping about in a chicken suit, clucking and pecking at the ground. This image cam impress your subconscious that person really isn't so special.

2. If the person is a drinker, recall now that their brain has been whittled down to the size of a walnut

6. If this offense is so great those two tricks aren't working, use your "Drop the curtain!" Trick. See the curtain rapidly unrolling to cover them. Turn off the lights in the theatre.

Then go practice one of your new akills:

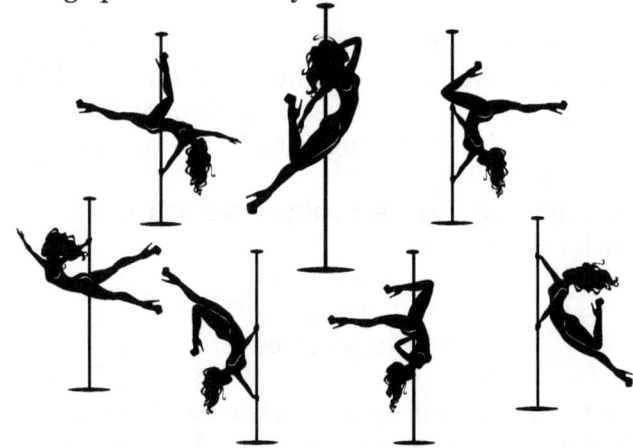

The Good News about a critical over-drinker: He gives you many opportunities to practice your new tricks. That means you'll learn these tricks—fast, to pop up when needed reflexively.

Practice: Write one negative thing the drinker (or other negative person) has said to—or about—you, and let it be something that hurt or angered you.

1. _____

_____

ANOTHER ONE! NOW!

2. _____

_____

For each hurtful negative thing that anyone says or has said, go back through your life to find just one example of your doing something different from what they are saying.

This is another trick akin to Thought-Switching that actually alters memories. It probably alters their vividness and importance more than the memory itself.

Your most harmful critic is yourself.

Nagging at yourself damages you worse than someone else's comments. It is especially severe when you repeat it, say or think it more than once. As you have seen, that is precisely the formula for making an idea become stronger. Want to become a real stumblebum? Just say out loud, "Oh, I'm so clumsy!" a time or two and it becomes truth.

Sometimes you say these things as a shield before someone else does—because that would hurt so bad and embarrass you so badly. Problem is, when you say it, it has a fast track and gets in deeper than when others do, so readjust your idea that saying something negative about yourself first, before anyone else can, is a good thing. It is not.

It's that sad child inside you, the one who believed she had to earn love by being perfect, by living up to what others demanded of her. She's the one who hangs onto these words; she was smart and she thought that if she beat herself with the criticism, it would make her do better! Give her credit, her motives are A+. She's just been aiming at a target that turns out to be the opposite of what she thought. She never knew until now that she was actually creating the likelihood that she would again stumble and appear clumsy. as her subconscious conformed to what she was saying about herself. And all of this has been because she wanted that person to love her! She thought that if she accused herself, the other person would see that she was on top of becoming perfect and would like her more. Who knows whether they will; probably not. The point is the person who really counts in the struggle for improving is the girl inside you, that intelligent, quick-witted girl being your subconscious.

Now pat her on the butt and tell her what a good and smart girl she is! Do this often.

When upsetting incidents stick in your mind, the Thought Switch is an effective technique.

Use it. When a memory is hurting, tune in to another station. Don't try to shut something down, just replace it; slide in something different.

> **Psych Note**: Nothing damages your self-esteem more than your own low opinion of yourself.
>
> Each time you think something bad about yourself pumps up a stronger sense that you are inferior.
>
> Research has shown that when you think and feel that you are inferior—inadequate—the mental belief takes on a life of its own. From pre-schoolers to Ph.D candidates, the results are the same: If you criticize the person prior to their doing some task, they will perform poorly.
>
> Boom!
> Got it?

Points to Ponder

The things drinkers say to their women are basically the same from drinker to drinker. That's how we know it's coming from an altered brain. Would you trust an airline pilot with an altered brain? A bus driver? Well, take back control of your soul and don't trust a mean mouth to be any different—and stay that way.

Don't open the door to anyone with an altered brain to play around inside your head, or take to heart their negative judgements of you. The more often you've taken in a negative comment about yourself, the deeper it will have gone, so some of the imbedded ideas will take more refuting than others. Just know this: Every time you talk back to a negative opinion about you, you strengthen your subconscious protective shield and boost your emotional strength. It's a magnificent payoff for learning a simple technique.

As you learn, be patient with yourself. As patient as you would be with a precious friend (which you are now becoming to yourself).

(Note: Einstein wrote that he sometimes did things he later thought were really stupid! (I mean, really! If even Einstein had stupid moments, how can you expect to never have one!)

Psych Note: Just who would use one of our human imperfections to beat you down? You can be sure of this: It will not be anyone who really loves you.

Those who really love you will find ways to tell you negative things that don't belittle you, don't make you feel inferior, stupid, worthless.

Those who really love you will find ways to teach you better ways, or suggest remedies and offer to help.

Those who really love you will not be smug after criticizing you.

A New Move

1. When (not "if") you are in the wrong, simply acknowledge what you did wrong and apologize!

2. Do not defend it or excuse yourself. Hold your tongue. Do not call yourself dumb. (After the apology, you can explain, but try to excuse the error. You may have a justified defense, but wait until after you've apologized, so any bother the incident has caused the person to calm before you offer any defense. Later is fine too.)

3. Do what you can at the moment to correct the situation.

4. Stretchy 'Em and Move Along.

* * *

Healthy Way to Handle Making an Error Trick

If you are responsible for a problem, use the experience in a positive way, as a builder.

1. Examine the actual error, not necessarily all the other person says it is.

2. Mentally do a quick search of your memory for something in the event that you might do better next time.

3. Visualize yourself doing it the new way. (This is a legitimate practice of the new way.)

4. Thought-Switch to a fun thing, or to feeling good about some good quality you possess.

5. Each time it comes back to mind, repeat steps 1-4.

Make a mental note of what you can do better when you do this next time, remembering the event not to beat yourself down but to keep getting better.

You, my darlings, are princesses, all of you, loved by God and likely once loved by the man who now assails you. You can only judge whether there is love in him today by his behavior today. No matter what he says to the contrary, any behavior that harms you physically, emotionally, or mentally is not coming from love. You cannot fall back on the "Oh, but I know he loves me" idea. Love doesn't do harm, especially intentional harm. And yes, he knows full well that the things he says hurt you.

You've heard it many times: Actions speak louder than words. Freud, the "master psychiatrist" tells mental health professionals, even today, that we must pay attention to a person's words, but remain just as attentive to their behavior.

He taught, over 100 years ago, that behavior is the best proof of words. Or dis-proof.

Following this 100-year-old wisdom, indispensable to professionals today, shows you exactly where you stand with others, no matter what they say. If their behavior doesn't match their words, write off their words!

You won't go wrong by believing the behavior; you got where

you are by believing others's words.
You can tell them so.
Or not.

The love you long for, and hang in with a bad relationship waiting for, does not exist in bad behavior. If that is made clear once, and the bad behavior continues, you can be sure that, no matter what his words say, there is no real love. Attraction, need, maybe—but no love. And anything short of love can't fill your need. Cut your losses here.

Just do it safely (see Chapter 9).

Love consists of caring for the welfare and happiness of the beloved. But you can't give that kind of love indefinitely without getting plenty of it in return. The major reason most drinkers's women hang in is their belief he will straighten up—sometime in the future. That he will finally appreciate them, value them, love them, treat them kindly.

But here's the problem: A man with bad behavior doesn't have much—or any—love to give. It won't ever come because it's not in there.

He has wants, needs, dependencies, and other selfish feelings, but love, the love you long for, just isn't there. If he ever *had* real love, alcohol destroys the brain cells that monitor and control how he thinks about and acts toward others.

Being needed (or used) is not being loved. Being needed is a minor need in the human, while being loved (and safe) are top priority needs. Consider that, even if he wants you because you do so much for him, is that how you really want to be loved?

It's certainly not the love you have a right to, the love you deserve, or the love that fills human needs.

Rebuilding Your Self-Confidence

Your self-confidence will grow like a well-tended garden as you gradually begin to drop away from negative people, at least limiting the time you must spend with them, and begin to associate only with nurturing people. How can you heal when you are still being shot at regularly? Would you take a wounded soldier who is just beginning to heal and throw him back into the heart of battle? Well then, don't do that to yourself.

Only you can protect the whole of who you are. If you must associate with critical people (boss, parent perhaps), make your contact as short as possible: Arrive late, leave early. Keep a heavy mental curtain to drop in a Thought Switch on cue.

For those of you who have been deeply hurt, know that after you've built up some strength, you will better deal with stressors; *no one* can do that well early on. Does anyone jump up off a sickbed and do jumping jacks? Completely heal after surgery? Consider this and be gentle with yourself.

Give yourself permission to take whatever time it takes to "do better." Your daily assignment is to be as kind and patient and protective of yourself as you are of others in your care. It's only when a wound is fully healed that it no longer is sensitive.

Healing takes time. Sometimes days, sometimes years. It takes what it takes and trying to force it actually rips the wound apart again, sometimes making you start the healing process all over again.

> **Psych Note:** The message you force into your subconscious when you push yourself is this: "You are inadequate so you must push yourself!" This reinforces low self-esteem and confidence. Stop it!

When controllers and bullies are refuted in any way, they either lash out verbally, or push you away. The way they handle being refused what they want depends on what they have learned about what puts pressure on you.

Clamped Lips and Move Along are your trick.

Okay, it's time to list three more good things about yourself. That will make nine! Recall the six things you listed earlier, and write them, then come up with three more. If you blank out, refer to this list, a few of the good things I know about you:

You are intelligent, caring, strong, talented, persevering, generous, helpful, understanding, patient (until you're not anymore), giving—and that's only for starters. Don't make me make the full list; the book would go on and on and on and on.

Let's put the whole list on the same page:

Nine Good Things I Know About Me

1. _____

2. _____

3. _____

4. _____

5 _____

6. _____

7. _____

8. _____

9. _____

A Magical Self-Healing Trick

Whatever qualities you list are the real you. You've been searching for her: here she is. Her very essence is made up of these wonderful qualities. This is who you are.

1. Read aloud all six of these good things you have listed.

2. Next, read them out loud slowly, thoughtfully, with feeling.

3. Now consider each quality, its beauty and value, and acknowledge again that you indeed have that quality.

4. Think about how much you like other people who have that good quality.

5. Bring that liking feeling onto yourself as you envision yourself with the quality you value.

No matter how down-hearted you may become (and remember, it's normal to sometimes feel down), you are still the spunky gal you remember, you still possess every good quality you once had. (Qualities are like blue eyes or brown eyes; you can appear to change them by wearing colored contact lenses, but they're still really blue or brown or whatever.)

She's still there. She hasn't gone anywhere. Best of all, she's starting to itch—itching to get back into action!

Having fun, feeling good about herself!

Enjoying.

Laughing.

* * *

So—Are You Really Alone?

The drinker's woman feels alone because she has been, likely for quite a while—even when he was there. She is not alone in the problems we're working on here. You may not see all those millions of other women out there who right now are grappling with exactly the same stresses. That doesn't mean they're not there. (You probably can't see Atlanta from where you are either. That doesn't mean it's not there!)

The feeling of being alone, that no one would understand you and that others will judge you is common—but that doesn't mean those beliefs are justified. No matter how unique you may feel, you aren't. Based on those National Institutes of Health findings, as many as 30 million U.S. women are in a relationship with a man who is drinking too much, or are scarred by the past relationship with one. Wounds, scars cause problems, create stress.

The United States has roughly 300,000,000 citizens. More than half of them, around 200,000,000, are of drinking age or drinking. More than half of drinkers, around 110,000,000, are male. One landmark National Institutes of Health survey found that as many as one in three, 33 percent of drinkers, admit that they drink more than the "safe" amount (the amounts you saw earlier, one beer = one ounce of alcohol—that list.

Drinking more than the safe level means they are "over-drinking." What do you think makes more than that "not safe"?

Right! It's the amount where cell damage is measurable.

More than half of adult Americans drink, and this survey indicates that as many as a third of them admit over-drinking. As you have seen, for a drinker to admit he's drinking more than the safe level is a miracle—and it's likely that nearly as many didn't give the honest answer.

In any case, we're talking about millions of over-drinkers,

99.9 percent of them having had many more than one intense relationship. And that accounts for more women who have been affected by the bad behavior of over-drinking men.

(Other NIH studies report that the number of over-drinkers is on the rise, and that means the percentage of the population that drinks and over-drinks are also rising.)

My point (that I make repetitively!): Lots and lots and lots of other beautiful women—very much like you—suffer in much the same way. You are not alone in your confusion or misery.

Oh, did you say that you don't see any of those other women?

Well, of course you don't! That's because they're just as good at hiding their situation as you have been, darlin'.

In addition to all these women who are just in the United States, newspaper articles from around the world—England, Scotland, Ireland, Australia, Thailand, China, many African countries, and more—all report similar statistics and problems with over-drinking. Women solidly packed around the world.

When we add to the number of current women with over-drinkers at least as many more, double their number, what do we have? It likely doubles these numbers. Most over-drinkers have many failed relationships behind them, and in all those relationships, they were behaving at some level of the same disorder. All of those women have been wounded similarly.

Without help of some kind, these women, your true spiritual sisters because they have similar special qualities, lives and personalities changed for the worse.

The Good News: A qualified psychotherapist can address and remedy most of this damage and, if she's savvy, can do so it in a short time.

Some of these millions of women got out of their relationships by breaking up, running away, divorcing; some were freed when the over-drinker finally died of alcohol-associated illnesses, or was killed in an accident, or in a fight, or one of alcohol's physical destructions, or he was one of the many who eventually commit suicide. (I know. Let's don't comment here.)

And many of these women, wounded, maybe hardened, got out of their relationships in one of the most painful ways: The over-drinkers left them for someone else.

Imagine a woman who has been mentally and emotionally

beaten down, frightened for her safety, her self-worth and self-confidence almost nonexistent, who is still trying to prove she is worthy of love. She has been told she is a shrew (a nice word for what is probably said), she's ugly and a mess, that she's crazy and a bitch, and that now he has found someone better than her.

Does she need caring, tenderness, information?

That woman needs all the information you can give her! By all means, pass along this book—while assuring her that you can relate. Tell her that the harms done to a drinker's woman stay with her even after the drinker is gone. Just like the hole is still in the body after the leaves.

A substantial number of these women turn to alcohol themselves, or to drugs or prescriptions to dull their mental and emotional pain. Now you know that many of the tricks here have the power to do that for them. Pass along what you learn; you have the power to rescue them.

It is common for a drinker to have (and hide from prospective lovers) a long list of failed relationships. For many, there will be a trail of wounded women, used up and dumped. And blamed for all the problems.

What's amazing is that, up to the very end stage, these quite often mean or disgusting men can still act so cute or funny or romantic that they convince a new woman that they're a good catch! (Quite likely you heard all about the crazy ex-wife when you met this guy.) These men convey to new prospects that their earlier relationships ended because of some terrible flaw in the woman!

In most cases, the sweet soul that falls for such advances is a lot like you; she thinks, "Oh, he just needs love. I know I can love him enough to heal him." You know, just you may have.

It's only a matter of time before the new ones are in exactly the same situation (and shape) as the last one (you). While she may have thought poorly of you early on, she'll soon begin feeling compassion and sympathy as she sees the real guy—the one that you know won't be able to keep his "nice" on for long.

(Note: It's not uncommon for the exes of over-drinkers to become friends after the new one's reality sets in.)

Again you may ask, "If there are so many, why don't I see them?"

The sad part: Most will not heal without outside help.

Why She Hides
   The drinker's woman believes that if others knew the truth of what goes on at her house, or what has been going on, they would judge her harshly.
   She believes they will blame her for being a bitch, or stupid, or think she is weak and crazy. Sometimes she keeps her silence for his sake; she doesn't want to shame him or lose his job. She doesn't want him to get in trouble because of the fall-out on her and children. Most over-drinkers are so good at acting like they are okay, their women have already discovered that few people believe them when they do talk about it. He's a master at slipping blame onto others in order to come across as a victim. She, on the other hand, dodges being thought of weak and helpless (some women love it, but rarely a drinker's woman). Or crazy.
   Most fear they really are crazy, so they hide away. Living with an over-drinker and his behavior creates the same kind of wounds in their women. The only good thing about that is that they understand each other.

   Financial security isn't worth abdicating your soul.
   Or your health.
   Or your potential, and a positive future.
   Or your wonderful Inner Child, Inner Actress, Inner Princess, and all the rest of the gang.

   Bouncing back requires beginning to talk to someone who understands, who really understands; take care to choose only those people you trust to keep your secrets (or those who are legally bound to secrecy—such as a minister, priest, rabbi, physician, therapist, or attorney) and Alanon women. Be mindful, however, that in most states, if you tell a doctor, nurse, or therapist that your partner is violent, that he hits you, they are legally bound also to report it or lose their license to practice their livelihood.
   I tell you this not to prevent your being honest with your helper, but to prepare you for the possibility she must call in others to help with your situation. While most professionals praise the purpose of this requirement, we see its downside. As yet, we have no other answer in sight.
   One encouragement: Together, we women and professionals have the power to fix such glitches. When women band together,

around a women's shelter or the need for one, or the need for changes in laws, they have consistently brought all the positive changes in the law and in cultural thinking that we have going for us now. You have the power to become one more link in a chain that has been changing the world. The education of women, especially in their personal worth and rights to life, freedom, and the pursuit of happiness.

Since you need to begin talking to someone about your experiences and your work on changing your life, you have an opportunity to practice another new skill: This skill is like sticking your toe in the water before jumping in.

Just as with all the people you encounter, including potential lovers, with a therapist you carefully assess and test her before entrusting *anything* to her. You get practice maintaining an emotional distance sufficient to keep from being taken in.

You want to believe the best of people, but you have already learned that not all are worthy of that confidence. Much as you hate that truth, you now are accepting it—just like the lucky girls who had savvy teachers have done before you.

Even if the person is a professional, check their reaction to lesser parts of your story before you throw open your life's doors to the down and ugly. If the professional fails your test by showing any signs other than caring and acceptance, practice your new and growing skill of assertiveness if you can—tell her what has scared you off. She may be unaware. But if you're not there yet, just finish your session, or end it there; thank her, and leave. You are learning to take care of yourself.

Fearing others's judgements keeps many women silent when opening up could be their salvation. Move Along and find another person or professional to test for working with.

What Most Women Need at This Point
What most women seem to need is a way to put distance between themselves and the over-drinker for enough time to regain their mental and emotional balance. Perhaps long enough to also begin making plans for any changes they want to make when they return. Or plans to stay away.

No, you don't have to leave him.

If you think it's best for you and your interests to stay with him, and there is absolutely no danger of violence, you may be able to do that.

Indeed, some women have picked up this information and their bags of new tricks, and been able to live relatively well with their drinker.

Still, getting some space from him is necessary to look at your options with a clear mind, which you can't have as long as you are in a stressful situation. Some women have been able to get away from the drinker briefly (or forever) under the guise of visiting family for a few days. (Be aware that many drinkers will welcome her leaving, especially if she doesn't let on she needs to be away from him. They will welcome the freedom to do as they wish—as if they aren't doing that now.)

BUT—

If your drinker is, or has *ever* been, violent, or has ever threatened you about what he'll do if you leave him, **you must go to Chapter 9 before planning any absence.** Most of the 2,000 women blatantly killed by their partner this year will either try to leave without very good help, or mentally dismiss his possible potential to harm them. Most of those 2,000 murders of beautiful women come either while she's trying to leave, or shortly after she does.

Just to threaten to leave him can put the life of many in danger. Your makeup doesn't want to believe this. Thus, we are murdered right and left and the murderer goes free or just serves a short term. Usually because he convinces a judge or jury that she was a bitch and egged him on and it was al her fault that he killed her.

When you consider how many women are killed annually by their partner, you must think beyond that, about those who have died in automobile wrecks while he was driving after drinking, and those not dead but only crippled, or scarred horribly—by knife, hot grease in the face, and hundreds of other horrors I've seen, heard about, and experienced. *This is not a trivial matter and you cannot approach it lightly. Your life may well hang in the balance, even if he has never been violent or threatened it.*

Furthermore, do not underestimate the drinker's need to control what you do, nor underestimate how he may react if he feels the threat of your leaving. *This bad response will happen even if he doesn't like you anymore! It's not about love; it's about control, and his ego. His manhood is being publicly criticized, in his understanding.*

Try not to do anything until you've talked with a qualified

counselor, preferably a woman who is well trained in these situations. That's because leaving and planning to leave are the most dangerous times, when most women killed by their partner are killed. Such women are reliably found on the hot lines at a woman's center, as well as professional counselors. (No—there is no "safe" separation from a controlling or abusive over-drinker, even if he appears to be nice about it. You must maintain your guard. Remember too, it's better to pretend you still love him than to have him become violent. Do or say whatever you need to when you are protecting your safety.)

While controlling men might not allow your visiting family, visiting friends or family can give you a break for examining your alternatives. You can always set the visit for a day or two, then call and extend the time later. While there is a good time to set up safety counseling. You can call any women's center and talk to anyone answering the phone without fear of being overheard or traced. They either will talk with you or set you up with someone else. Professional counselors are available in almost every part of the country today; they all have information on safety planning and available services for women.

The woman you talk to when you call a women's center is almost always a volunteer who has survived and moved on, perhaps even using local shelter services. They serve as a volunteer now, wanting to pay back for what they received. (Indeed, I have a mental picture of you in the future being in that seat yourself.)

I shy away from guiding you to a minister outright. Many will understand and support you, but some of them will insist you remain in an abusive marriage because they believe it is a sin to escape bad treatment, that husbands are to be the master of wives—as some scripture instructs.

Many a woman has been sent home from a conference with her minister having been told, "God says you must stay with the man! He is your master! Go back and follow God's commands on this." And they have been punished, maybe beaten, when the husband found out they had dared to go talk to anyone. Many, many women. I was one of them.

You must be careful to whom you entrust your secrets. Better to be too careful than to err in a way that will get you hurt.

As to ministers, it's also true that many more have begun

giving women help in escaping an abusive (or drunkenness) situation. If you don't know his stance on this issue, check with the minister's secretary or assistant *if she is trustworthy* and ask or feel her out about how he handles this kind of situation before opening yourself to him. This may be my personal bias, as I suffered a great deal from what I was told and counseled to do by ministers. But that was a long time ago.

Should you think that you're weak for being in this situation, consider that other women facing the same have become at least as rattled and disintegrated. Especially if they had been betrayed and mistreated, badgered or threatened, bullied or cheated on, lied to and disrespected.

Here's your mantra:

Whatever shape you are in is precisely what would exist in any other (similar) woman in your situation.

The lucky girls who were raised to *know* how to avoid pitfalls may not have much compassion for your case, so don't be surprised if you run into that. I certainly have. Just keep your contact with those you suspect are that type to a minimum.

Your condition is not due to being weak, darlin'. In fact, it's from being too strong. Staying in a situation where other women would have folded long ago. Whether others see that or give you credit for it, it is your truth.

If it's best (and safest) for you to stay with him now, you can use your new perspective and new tricks to ease dealing with both him and events. Many other women have done so, most not for long though. I suggest that, to make all of this easier, at your earliest opportunity you look up your local Alanon and call them. Make contact. Talk only as much as is comfortable; they will understand when you feel like you need to stop or get off the phone. Tell only what you are comfortable with sharing now; you don't need to tell everything.

You don't need a sponsor to become an Alanon, they are Add-ons later. Just go to a meeting and tell them you need help and support. Your sponsor will be a woman you meet at an Alanon meeting; it may take a month or so of looking for a good fit. She'll be a woman you get along with and admire, one you want to be more like. That's your winner. Except in dire cases, most any Alanon will consent, gladly becoming your teacher and best friend—just as I hope you do for another frightened or confused woman in the future.

Strengthen your return to life by calling a friend or family member you were close to in the past. Rebuild as many of your nurturing relationships as you can, but do it slowly. Some of those relationships may not be as nurturing as you thought. List three people who are possibilities here. (And you don't have to tell them much to get the relationship going again. Only that you've had problems *and that you have missed them!*)

1. _____

2. _____

3. _____

Some of your old friends may have felt hurt if you pulled away. Now you can tell them how difficult it was for you to continue in your friendships, but don't belabor it. How bad you felt, depressed, hopeless, whatever. Some people may not accept your reasons. Their hurt feelings can cause them to be less than welcoming when you first make contact. Even so, understanding this and being prepared for it, you won't crash. If they back off, just tell them you understand how they must feel, and that you really hope they'll change their minds—that you'll be waiting. (I frequently hear that in a few days, the person who originally rejected renewing a friendship called back, apologized, and set up a lunch date!)

If they don't call you back, follow up anyway; give it a week or two, then contact them again. If that one still "isn't available," move on to other names on your list. (Most women who've done this report that almost all of their old friends told them how much they missed them and happily renewed the friendship. Actually, most people figure out what's been going on.)

Setting Free Your Inner Princess

One mental trick that will change your life is adopting that law of Bad News always holds some Good News. I'm not talking about mass disasters or death of a loved one: I'm talking about most of the Bad News that comes into your everyday life. Bad News almost always has some positive element—brings along something that can be turned to good. And that is your Good News. By searching for if needed, and latching onto the Good

News that is always part of a Bad Event, I guarantee you will change your life. You will establish a strong basis for any changes you want to make. Every time the ugly splatters, you get a new opportunity to practice this habit. Consequently, you may as well start thinking of his ugly stuff as always carrying something you can take as positive, the Good News.

Being stuck on Bad News cripples you; it fills your body and brain with the chemicals that encourage confusion and despair. It builds stress upon stress. Coming up with even a simple positive possibility in a bad situation primes your inner pump with positively charged chemicals. It's often an immediate lift to even consider doing it.

Even in a disaster, you can make yourself focus on all those around you who are helping each other, the goodness that still lives in the hearts of so many. And if they're not already at work helping, you get busy and get them started! This is your new life direction. Once you begin this new way of meeting negative events, your subconscious—ever your friend—latches onto it and makes it a firm habit. That thinking rapidly becomes your new reflex because it brings such intense rewards—and you know what a pig your subconscious is for rewards!

* * *

The 'Stay vs. Separate' Question

Some of you to will be able to stay with your guy, but aim for that only if it's what you believe is best for you. (You may have a struggle beginning to be a little bit selfish.) The cure is always to remember that if you're not okay, nothing and nobody else in your life will be okay either.

In some cases a woman can stay with the drinker and become reasonably happy by using the tactics here and those you'll learn as you advance—in therapy or Alanon or similar. The only time you must leave is if he is violent. Yes, and that's based on the high number of women killed and severely injured (burn scars over their bodies, health gone due to multiple stabbings, and suicide are examples). While leaving can be a dangerous time, and the difficulties of getting help in planning and whatever else is needed, it's still better to be safe. Be safe now and live to reconsider later.

If you stay for your children's sakes, you may unknowingly be harming them. Here's how: Children use the adults around them as models for the way to live and behave. Their major source of personality formation comes from watching, then imitating, their parents.

Many a child has vowed never to become like the failing parent, yet all that he or she has absorbed will still shape their personalities, and their thinking about male and female roles. And many, many of those children will go on to also over-drink and ruin their lives.

The same child who belittles her mother for what she sees as weakness is likely to get hooked up with the same kind of man. Believe it.

That's because this kind of man is what is being imprinted on her "picker" as what men are like.

Sons are watching in the same way and absorbing the drinker's behavior and attitudes toward most everything. As a result, your precious little boys are very likely to imitate the thinking and behavior they see in him.

On the other hand, however, some research finds that children whose mothers pointed out the wrongness of the man's behavior, then gave them substantial reasons for their staying with him, rarely had the same bad outcomes. This means that if you choose to stay, be sure to have these talks—more than once—with your children.

Contrary to what society tells us, your telling a child that a misbehaving dad loves them but he just has an illness is a disservice to the child. The child who is told those things learns that people can treat you badly, ignore you, even hurt you, but still believe that they love them anyway. This may be what you learned.

Some never get the chance to learn that love means you don't behave badly toward those you love.

> **Psych Note:** Girls "take it" because they believe that even if the guy is bad or mean to her, he loves her. Boys learn to be the way they observed, expecting their woman to know they love them anyway.

Tell your children the truth, that dad has used a legal drug so much it has damaged parts of his brain, causing his behavior to go bad. **Do not say, "But he loves you,"** not unless he actively and regularly shows them his love. Otherwise, they absorb the

idea that people can love you but treat you badly, or ignore you.
Some of you absorbed those concepts.

Unless you intervene, children will come to expect men to behave the way they see their father behave, and women to behave the way they see their mother behave. Children may verbally reject some of what they see, but the over-drinker's children frequently slide into similar unhealthy relationships.

A boy swears he'll never be a drunk like his father. I have heard hundreds of men say that was how they thought when they watched their fathers—yet they became alcoholic and confess publicly that they behaved as badly as the man they watched.

A girl will swear she'll never let a man hit her or treat her the way her dad treats her mom, but she is still set up by her early imprinting to be attracted to, even comfortable with, a guy who has many of the same traits that were part of her father's personality. That's because they will be familiar to her. Some of you got where you are that way too.

I generally don't recommend separation unless there is violence. I make sure every woman knows that I'm all for separating if there is violence. Domestic Abuse, like alcoholism, doesn't appear to change for the better. It just gets worse.

When some batterers get old, they may to stop. But what's happened to that woman living in his creation of hell?

Research shows that mental and emotional abuse are almost as destructive mentally and emotionally as physical abuse. I also recommend taking care of yourself—good care of yourself. Don't wait for someone else to do it.

While I'm sure it has happened, I've never seen children of a drinker's woman be more seriously harmed by their parents's separation than what I've seen come to most when parents don't separate. (The sad part is that staying together was probably done for the sake of those children.)

That isn't to say they won't suffer any harm from separation; what I'm saying is that I've never seen the damage to a child's sense of who he or she is and becomes, be greater than the damages they receive from staying. A solid, healthy marriage is certainly the best atmosphere for children to grow and learn. The chaotic, scary or closed environment of an over-drinker's home is not a snug nest for raising healthy children.

On the other hand, if your home environment isn't too

destructive to you or them, the information and tricks in this book can begin equipping you (and them) to stay where you are and build happier and healthier lives for yourselves.

Do not tell your children their father loves them if he doesn't act like it!

Don't try to ease their pain by saying that their father loves them. That is defining love as including bad treatment.

Instead, focus them on their own wonderful qualities and talk to them about real love. Point any examples you have seen in them—being there for one another, helping and caring about others, wanting to spend lots of time together, hugs and kisses. Talk to them about how successful they will be because of those beautiful qualities they have.

Teach them that bad treatment is the opposite of good treatment, and the absence of good treatment. You now are your children's healthy role model. What you accomplish with honesty now, even though painful, may be one of the greatest gifts you will ever give them.

If you are contemplating leaving, and are not sure if that is best for you, this simple bit of work with five steps may help settle at least some of your issues. I call this The Go, or No-Go Decision Guide, and you'll find it on the following page.

The Go, or No-Go Decision Guide

1. Draw a line down the middle of a regular-size sheet of paper.

2. On one side, at the top, write "Go," and "No Go" over the other.

GO	NO GO
_____	1._____
_____	2._____
_____	3._____
_____	4._____
_____	5._____

3. a) Under "Go" list all the reasons you can think of for separating.
    b) Under "No Go" list all the reasons you can think of for staying.

4. Next, scrutinize each item on each list and assign each one a number from 1-10, where 1 means it's not very important to you, and 10 meaning it's life-or-death important.

5. Compare the columns and weights. Take some time to think about it. Make any changes that come to you as you consider the problem: add items, change points, whatever.

Discuss what you find with a trusted friend or counselor to be sure you aren't fooling yourself on some of your points. You are free to change whatever you think needs to be changed.

Having made your Go/No-Go chart and pondered it, you are in a better position to make your best decision.

A bonus for making and working on this list is that decisions made this way rarely come back on you to make you doubt yourself. When they do, you always have the black-and-what facts you based your decision on, and you will always again agree with that decision. And you can re-do this exercise at any time, any number of times. All anyone can do when making decisions is her very best with the information available at the time.

No matter what you decide, you'll know, remember, that you used the best reasoning available to you at the time it needed to be made.

What's comes next?

Daily Increasing Your Care for Yourself

You demand a lot of yourself, yet I have observed that most of you do little to keep the machine you demand so much of in good shape. (If you're waiting for him to change before you think you can start on your own changes, you may go to your grave before he does.)

Experience with over-drinkers has shown that it takes something truly awful happening to them before they even consider changing. And it takes time, sometimes a very long time. Alcohol gives them so much, and to them the price is always worth it. Only a powerful reason is enough to make them surrender. And what would be a powerful reason to him? It has to be something that hurts him—terribly. The longer he continues over-drinking, the more awful that event will have to be to overcome his growing need to drink. (And recall that he's steadily working with fewer and fewer brain cells.)

First of all for you, understand that important event can never happen if you are shielding him in any way.

It takes from five to twenty years for a man developing a problem with drinking to get to the ugly end, where he finally considers getting help (without which almost no one has *ever* made it). And the chance that his most determined efforts will work are practically nil.

Given that and all else you're learning, here's my question: *Are you willing to spend the next five to twenty years of your best self you'll ever have on the extremely slim possibility that he'll get better?* And stay that way?

If, and only if, staying with him is important for your own best interests—then do it (until it's no longer in your best interest.)

The most glaring idea is that you don't base your future

welfare on a fantasy that everything will one day be fine.

Finally getting to the point where he's entirely ready and willing to change (and do whatever it takes to stay that way), the five to twenty years it took to get to this point is still only the beginning, especially for you. There will be no true or deep changes for months, and only then if he keeps to his requirements.

Should he be one of the rare few who make the turn-around, it will take months for you to get much back. He also will need to work on the many changes he *must* make every day for the rest of his life in order for it to stick.

Even if he does *all* these things, recovery of all the things you want him to be cannot be banked on.

Getting through all it takes to get a man to treatment has been the focus of books for their partners until now. What they have not told you is that just getting to costly treatment doesn't mean he will straighten up—and if he does, it doesn't mean he will stay that way. Just completing treatment gives you absolutely no promises that he can or will stay "better." You must consider your own levels of strength and commitment.

Sadly, I've seen many marriages fall apart after a man finally got treatment and began a firm recovery. Seems odd, not to make sense for a woman to hold on through thick and thin while he was smashing everything in their lives, but then—when he goes into what looks like recovery—she leaves. But that's just the way it seems on the surface.

Why do you think these marriages and relationships fail so miserably after enduring so much? Here's why:

The changes the drinker's woman is looking for, has been dreaming of for years, don't come. Or, if they come, they fall away again. His important inner changes can require years to take root and stabilize.

With the diagnostic guidelines on over-drinking that are in use now, and "treatment" (in too many cases just an expensive fairy tale) being such as it is now, few over-drinkers will ever get what treatment is needed before it's too late to do any good. All of that must change, and drastically, if more than the few, the 6 to 10 percent who make it and stay straight, are to build new lives.

After all her years of hard work, the drinker's woman is crushed because she believed that treatment would bring back her Prince. Oh, he may peek out now and then, but it's not that same guy you hoped for. And out of the very few who will make it, even fewer will become the better part of themselves again—and stay that way.

Getting past the honeymoon stage following the man's entry into some form of treatment, a long-suffering woman discovers he's still stuck in many of his horsey-butt ways. And she is crushed. She can crack—or it feels like cracking. If this is you—don't collapse! Call out for help. It's available to you, instantly through Alanon. I know of no other channel on earth that can help women at this point.

Get help deciding on your next step. Avoid doing anything without thought and planning.

Why so many Similarities in Drinkers's Women?

Some people find it strange that drinkers's women are so similar. And they marvel that the mental and emotional wounds inflicted on them are so similar. Two facts explain this:

First, women's brains are wired in a special way. Women's brains differ from men's in over a hundred significant ways. What's more, women have important brain areas that men lack.

Women are wired to become attached to a mate who can help raise young, protect them all, and provide well for them. That explains having an eye for rich men. (While some interpret this tendency in women as greediness, that's all wrong. Women are wired to insure the survival of the human race. I've heard some men put women down for being "all about money." But even female animals look for a mate who will be a good provider and protector.) And good looks usually attest to good health, so women are wired to be swayed by good looks.

Another difference between men and women is that if a man loses his relationship, he can replace it easier than can a woman, especially if she has children. A break in a relationship can mean to a woman a break in having the basics needed for survival—a home, provision, protection, stability.

The result is that threats to a women's relationship generally arouse far stronger emotion than generally found in men. There emotional reactions stem more from their territorial instinct, but hers stem from the survival instinct.

Grasping these important physical and psychological differences between men and women, you must never again feel like a crazy woman for falling apart at threats to your relationship. You're wired that way, baby.

When men don't understand, don't be surprised. They don't even have the chunks of brain that contain this programming. They also are missing some of the brain areas that allow women to be able to empathize—to be sensitive to others's needs or pain. Men frequently make jokes or take potshots at this sensitivity in women. But the Manufacturer saw fit to program you this way.

Some Special Warnings

These differences turn out to make women far more vulnerable than men to the behaviors that over-drinking produces: harsh criticism, bullying, mean words, withdrawal, downfall of the home-nest, infidelity, abandonment If only emotionally.

Indeed, men flatly and swiftly leave relationships that have become as uncomfortable as yours has. You tend to stay because of your wiring, not because you're stupid. Actually, the man would have left this kind of behavior long ago.

> **Psych Note**: One study of the people entering treatment for alcoholism found that 80 percent of men still had a significant other. Only 20 percent of women did!

Just as people who suffer a stroke affecting the same parts of the brain tend to behave similarly, over-drinking causes over-drinkers to become more and more alike as they progressively get worse. Their brains are being affected in the same ways.

And this means that the wounds over-drinkers inflict on their women will be similar.

That's why you'll find so many kindred spirits in Alanon or ay codependent or similar group.

But look at the Good News hidden here: The similarities in personality and the experiences of drinkers's women means that they can form rapid and strong connections with each other, totally understanding each other like no one else can, or perhaps ever will. Their similarities create immense common ground. Their similar experiences also guarantee that neither will judge the other. They create supportive and nurturing friendships that last a lifetime. Indeed, it may be that other wounded-but-healing women are the only people who can ever truly understand you. I have found it to be so. The rest of the world just doesn't seem to "get" it.

One secret of living successfully with an over-drinker is to cease hoping for the Prince to come back and stay.

Another key: You absolutely must stop trying to fix him.

Don't even correct him anymore (unless he's hung-over and you're having "the talk"). You've already spent far too much of yourself at this useless activity.

After splitting with their over-drinker, many emotionally wounded women jump into a new relationship. (Yes, I did it too, so don't feel uniquely messed up if you have.) This happens because after horrible, even barely passable looks good.

Sadly, most of these relationships won't work; many become copies of the last one. And sadder still, most women will take that next relationship failure as one more proof of their inadequacy.

The major reason this happens is that the woman is still attracted to the same type of man that she was when this one caught her eye. Much like her over-drinker was at first: cute, funny, sweet, romantic.

Take this warning to heart: A relationship with a similar kind of man will have a similar ending.

When feelings begin to bloom, you must keep in mind your vulnerability due to your years of having your basic emotional needs unfulfilled. The need and hunger are so great that it is easy for a man who is just a nice guy, or who listens, or who is cute or funny . . . to take the reins in a new relationship. And it can seem like the perfect match.

Tragically, that's not the case. Why? Because you are still being attracted to the same kind of man. Think about it, keep track of it. You can block a growing emotion. The secret is not to feed it with fantasies—of lovemaking, or romantic moments, or sailing away forever to live happily ever after. Those thoughts and feelings are almost sure to arise the first few times you run into a man who is similar to the one you have now—in personality, interests, attitudes—and that similarity guarantees he will be very much like the one that isn't working out well.

You will have to begin learning more about yourself and what has been attractive to you in a man, and what traits in you set you up for a bad experience. Learn what they are, and I guarantee you that you can change them—sometimes in the flash of a moment. Often, when we suddenly realize what we are doing, or why we do things that way, it becomes a flash of change you feel throughout your entire body. And when that happens, it sticks!

DANGER! DANGER!

Reaching out to an understanding man at this point can have disastrous results. You are more vulnerable than you realize, and will be until you've healed and rebuilt. Needing someone, especially a man, to do that is a trap and can lead to terrible results. Here's why:

• You are in danger of a rebound effect. This is just your human wiring and the result of much wounding.

• You can easily fall in love with someone who is kind (yet not at all the partner you need).

• (PRIME DANGER!) The men you are drawn to at this point are likely to be similar to the over-drinker you're escaping.

Unless you've had counseling in that specific area, much of what attracts you is going to be the same, it's part of your formative thinking, but it ca be changed. It just takes a little time—and help from those who know the problem and its solution.

DANGER: If you follow your fancies early on, the outcome is likely going to be the same as what you have escaped.

The challenges of separating can cause a woman to reach out to another man for relief. She most surely needs some relief—attention and praise, compliments, warmth, laughter, and all the wonderful things a healthy relationship holds. And she will welcome reassurance that she is attractive. But until she does some work on what and who she's being attracted to and who is finding her attractive (often it will be someone looking for a "keeper," or "enabler," someone who will put up with him). That guy may love you to pieces the first couple of times you bail him out or kiss his booboo, but he is incapable of returning the kind of love you give, the kind of love you need, and the kind of love you deserve.

Work on changing many qualities in yourself are best and fastest done with a professional guiding you. Yes, it is expensive, but many therapists are willing to see you once a month, or even short sessions—in other words, in today's economy, many licensed therapists are willing to work with their clients.

I say you need outside help because we simply can't see ourselves accurately, and techniques you've used to change yourself may not have been any more successful than the techniques you've used trying to change him.

And if you don't find those weak spot in you and replace them with healthy new ways, your next relationships are quite sure to go the same way this one did.

You think that making up your mind to never to pick that kind of man again is enough, but it isn't. No more than him making up his mind not to drink is enough.

Very specific changes must be made—and those changes are almost impossible to make without qualified help. Trusting your inner self to even your best friend's psychological knowledge can be a big mistake—which is why therapists are taught not to ever work with people they are close to.

Besides, it's not a cookie-cutter approach that's needed. It must be tailored to the woman and the inner child who has made this journey with her.

Your subconscious settings as to what makes a man attractive are most likely broken. Good News: By the end of this book series (Book 2 coming soon, "Curing Codependent Quirks), you will see a huge change in yourself, how you behave with a man who is attractive to you, and what kind of man you are attracted to.

My personal experience coming through this self-searching and change (and others have told me they have experienced the same) is that qualities in a guy that used to turn me on have come to repel me. I emotionally and physically want to get away from them.

The follow-up book to this one guides you through examining various qualities of your personality and teaching you and giving you tricks to make needed adjustments. It is scheduled for publication in January 2016.

Awareness of your vulnerability now doesn't mean you must live without relief or comfort—or sex!

It means you understand that those good feelings are not true love.

While true love has lots of good feelings, good feelings are not necessarily true love. You can enjoy compliments, being liked and appreciated by another man, and you can have excellent sex—all you have to do is be aware your unfulfilled emotional needs will make you feel like you are a princess who has found her prince.

That is extremely unlikely.

Love, the kind that lasts, is a bond that grows over time. The initial, exciting, attraction is often and mistakenly called love. Some couples I've interviewed who have been married for over 25 years tell me that they were not at all attracted to each other in the beginning.

A tip-off that you're off to a bad start is that it feels like being "in love" from the start. From the first encounters. You have all kinds of fantasies. You're picking out your wedding dress.

Early good feelings are a cross between having fun with someone likely on his best behavior, and all your hot chemistry stirring. Your body wants to be held for emotional fulfillment (but that's so not enough! And your body wants, likely needs, sex and all your most wonderful brain chemicals are flowing.

Your being without tender love for so long, however, can set you up to be in something more like "heat" than in "love," the kind of relationship that grows and lasts.

A good motto: What begins as a flash usually ends in a crash.

Until you've made good progress in repairing and rebuilding your inner life and your picker settings, you can enjoy the company of men, but keep in the front of your mind how easy it is to form an attachment to someone who is good to you. So was this troubled man you have now, at first.

Until your picker has undergone a makeover, you can't help being attracted to someone much like the last one.

What appears attractive to us is built on impressions from our youngest years. And it doesn't change on its own.

Furthermore, you likely have been deprived of wonderful, wild, loving, gratifying sex; this makes you very vulnerable to feelings that can feel like "love." Do not ignore your sexuality, but don't mistake all that chemistry and excitement for love. It is not.

Being sexually attracted to someone isn't love. Enjoying sex isn't grounds for a lasting relationship.

Remember this: Even if you miss the mark on your first few tries (as I did), turn that Bad News into Good News: You can use each bad experience to learn something new about yourself, what has been attracting you, more areas of yourself you want to readjust. That opportunity is Very Good, and for some, well worth the not-so-hot experience.

Getting Honest with Doctors and Counselors

Picture a woman hunched over, arms raised over her head, a stricken expression, ducking and dodging. Let's say she is dodging a meteor shower, frantically looking this way and that to avoid being smashed, ducking and trying to find a safe place. Consider how she can appear to others. If someone observes her without knowing there's a meteor shower in her district, they may well determine that she must be mad.

And this is the way many drinkers's women have been judged, assessed, diagnosed. A counseling client is always diagnosed based on signs of mental disorders. (It's necessary if you use insurance; they won't pay without some kind of mental health diagnosis.)

The drinker's woman's way of avoiding harm is to stay on the alert every moment to prevent verbal attacks, explosions of rage. How do others interpret what they see in her? Even professionals can get it wrong. A woman can appear to be suffering from high anxiety. And she is, but it's not a mental disorder. She's suffering from the fatigue of dodging real meteors. When she runs out of steam, she collapses; she appears to be deep depression.

What's a professional to think?

Medication for either anxiety or depression: Often they take the edge off the stress of relationship changes, and I'm all for them when it's clear that is their sole purpose—and not a lifetime need.

The problem with the medications is that they do absolutely nothing to change the fall meteors, so your problem will not improve.

Working in specific ways toward simple inner changes can alter or halt negative feelings. Some of you may be genetically more susceptible to anxiety or depression. This is common enough. In that case, you may need a mild medication, perhaps for the rest of your life. It's like having an inherited vulnerability to diabetes or heart trouble. You are now committed to take as good care as ever you can of this precious woman (who is you) and her Inner Child.

The professional who prescribes medication must address the cause of anxiety and-or depression, help the client determine what life changes may be needed, then be wiling to help her plan, all the while working with her to rebuild her self-esteem, self-confidence, and the rest of her healthy self. You can see from this list why I so often recommend a trained and licensed professional to move you along. Short-term is fine—actually, preferable, for the kind of work you'll benefit most from. You will be able to do most of the work of putting you back together just fine on your own.

When you get stuck, something isn't changing after you give it the best you know, then go to a counselor for one single thing you want to change about yourself. Be clear with the professional what you are doing and she should jump right on board. If she fails to do that, perhaps you can try out other professionals until you find one who can work that way with you.

There's probably a lot in your past that could benefit from working through, but you can't get an overhaul all at once on this problem. You don't need to spend much time exploring the past except to unearth a few examples of things that could be associated with whatever you are specifically working on at the time.

After getting help with one issue, take a break. Return when you are ready to work on another issue that's not responding to your efforts..

Many excellent physicians and mental health professionals don't know that you live in a district of surprise meteor showers. They can only diagnose by what they see. They match what they see to a list of signs describing a specific disorder. They do this the same way a physician would match the signs of fever, aches, vomiting and diarrhea to flu, signs known to indicate of specific disorders.

Your signs may suggest anxiety disorder or depression, or both; almost all drinkers's women have both of these emotional-chemical swings, but what you suffer isn't a true anxiety disorder or a true depressive disorder. It's a reactive form of anxiety—or depression.

"Reactive" is the label we professionals apply to a disorder that is caused by a known precipitant, as opposed to just popping up or coming out of your head. You may exhibit every sign of chronic depression or anxiety, but it won't be true depression or anxiety; it's a reactive depression or anxiety. And the difference that separates reactive disorders is that treating the sufferer won't cure them until the triggering cause is removed. Only after removing the source of these problems can real treatment begin.

It can be very helpful as you begin working through your

situation, but do not think it's all you'll ever need. Medication can't fix the causative problem the way an antibiotic can fix an infection.

It's helpful to see a qualified, licensed counselor prior to talking to your physician about medication, because it is likely your physician settles for slight improvement, thinking of antidepressants and anti-anxiety medication like blood pressure medicine—something you'll just have to take for the rest of your life. In most of the United States, you can obtain both anti-anxiety and anti-depressant medications from your family physician; you don't have to see a psychiatrist, although most physicians are glad to have input from a mental health professional. Sign a release with your counselor so she can talk with your physician. This input enlarges your physician's understanding, then she can prescribe the best medications for your unique case.

For any help to be successful, you must tell the professional involved everything about your experience. They are professionals; they hear it every day; they do not judge their patients; they seek only to understand and then select the best remedies. If you perceive a professional person judges you as anything other than a beautiful soul she is blessed to be working with, get another professional!

Professionals can only treat you for whatever they think the problem is, based on what they know about you. If you hold back, out of embarrassment or shame, you block getting the best help.

Know Yourself

True anxiety, by definition, is having fear that isn't realistic.

That's not what is going on with you. Your fears are realistic for the most part, fear of very real threats, for example, your fear of him exploding without warning is absolutely realistic. *In a war zone, fearing being hit by a bullet is not called anxiety—it's a normal response to a real situation. It is rational fear. Do not allow anyone, professional, family, or general critic, to tell you that you are mentally disordered and suffer from a disorder. You suffer from a very real consequence of trauma!*

Should You Try to Get Him Into Treatment?

Many women ask if they should have their over-drinkers forced into treatment. Oh, yes, by all means—but only so long as you don't expect it to fix him. If you can afford it or arrange it, by all means do that. Just don't expect it to work—or at least, to work for long.

Most people think of treatment as if it's the solution—the cure, but now you know the dismal recovery rate of people who go to all forms of treatment. It's clearly not the miracle solution.

The drinker's woman has, in most U.S. states, the power to start proceedings to get her over-drinker into treatment, whether he's willing or not. But I've yet to see more than a handful of successes—out of hundreds. My reason for saying, "Yes, try to get him into treatment," is because you need the break! That time will give you time to regroup to some extent, and also to look for help and guidance about what to do next—for your welfare, not his!

This is why you should not go to an addictions counselor to get the deeper help you need for your own survival. See the treatment program's counselor if they are available to you because they can give you better understanding of what is going on with him. Just do not look for your cure there any more than you expect for a cure for him in Alanon.

You can hope, even pray, for his success, but do not base your life decisions on the belief that treatment will cure him. At its best, treatment in almost every case is still extremely wanting in its techniques, and extremely expensive, with no guarantees at all. Treatment programs will not publish their true "success" rate; what some publish is a rate based on—of all things—

- only three months after completion of treatment!
- what the over-drinker tells them over the telephone!

To make your task of getting help for him even more challenging is that only a sprinkling of treatment programs will give you any facts at all about the percentage of success in their program; even then, statistics can be swayed easily to say what their users want them to say. I learned the skills of creating research, which included what *not* to do. Turns out the what-not-to-do part is what, if you do it, will twist the outcomes of the research, will change their interpretation. You can only be sure of any statistics on treatment if they have been conducted by university-trained researchers, on grants not paid by invested corporations—and then, you must require more than just one outcome. If research isn't replicated, it is almost always worthless.

I keep looking, but have still only found that the treatments that give you "success" statistics have a strange definition of "success." You must dig to get the truth on this matter. It is common to label as success being three months, or six months, or even a year without a drink or drug. But as you are seeing, even that is no assurance at all that he will be okay tomorrow.

The worst part of this? Every single research I've investigated relies on what the drinker tells them—usually by telephone. Can't you just hear it now:

"Hello, Mr. Jones, this is your treatment program calling to see how you are doing."

"Oh, I'm doing just great!" he says.

"Have you had anything to drink since you left us?"

"Oh, no, no, no!"

Here, it can as easily be his denial kicking in as a genuine lie. If he has only had a little bit, a few times, he has dismissed them from being counted as "drinking." To him, he may not be lying. He defines "success" in yet another way.

Beware any claim of "success."

There is no such thing as "success" in alcohol treatment when success means stopping and staying stopped. In recovery, the people who make it know this and will tell you.

My own mentor informed me the day I reached my first year anniversary of being clean and sober: "Okay, do you know what comes next?" I stopped my strutting and crowing to say, "What?"

"A year and a day."

Reality: It's still just one decision at a time.

His reminder had its effect. Well, at least until now . . . .

This is a good time to go back to re-read the ideas you've listed in your Mastery exercises. See if you can already tell that some of these new ideas are showing up in your thinking.

* * *

**Next Page
The Easiest, Fastest, Never-Fail Trick Ever!**

The Easiest, Fastest Shut-Him-Up Trick
While living with a drinker, some rules for you will make your life much sweeter. When "discussions" between you and your drinker arise after around 6:00 p.m., and he's not willing to let it rest, this trick usually does the job you need done. It's the Shut Him Up Trick.

It has only one very simple, and for him, very delightful, step.

The Shut Him Up Trick
1. Go get him a cold beer (or pour him a drink), presented with a Stretchy-Lip Smile, say something about, hold up on that discussion for a moment while I do xyz (go to the bathroom?) Now you can either Move Along and forget to come back.

Or seduce him—if that's your fancy.

* * *

**Straight Talk About Life and Death—
And Crippling and Scarring**
Trying to be nice about his driving after even one drink won't work—except in his very early stage. It requires the assertiveness you'd show if he suddenly pulled out a blindfold and put it on, put the car in gear, and starting driving. How would you react then? Whatever it is, that's how you can act now.

Being nice about it is almost guaranteed to cause him to flare up and bulldoze you. You weather that simply by standing firm, not allowing anything he says to change anything—and holding your hand out for keys (or hiding them in the first place when you see him drinking).

Should all of that fail, firmly refusing to ride with him and following through has been very effective for many women.

Once she has to call a relative or friend to come get her, he knows his secret is out. He will surrender the keys to avoid being outed. Even though protesting creates difficulties for you, it's easier than losing a leg. Or a child.

A high level of assertiveness is required. And any licensed therapist can teach you assertiveness in one or two sessions.

One thing to bear in mind: If he's been drinking heavily, he won't remember any of it tomorrow—and what he remembers, he'll be ashamed of. So go ahead and be mean!

Be prepared for him to react like a HB. Struggle to speak in a normal tone—as if you're best buds.

Your priority, your first priority, is survival, not avoiding his wrath!

Your survival. Uncrippled. Unscarred. And your children's survival as well.

Upsetting him doesn't hold a candle in importance to those prospects.

Sometimes the lighter side is a good approach. Think how you'd say these things if he were stuffing himself with beans—eating huge bowls of beans all three meals a day—and insisting that you sleep with him? Would you just give up, stop protesting, surrender? Comply? Lay down and endure it?

How would you address the problem? Try to attach this example to thoughts of him driving after even one drink. Put a lightness in your voice as you first mention it to him.

Slip on that same attitude when he insists on driving after he's had more than one drink.

- State your intent to drive with calm assurance.
- If that fails, state clearly your determination to resist.

Or will you just settle into the passenger seat?

Learned Helplessness? Many a drinker's woman has been killed by it. Or crippled. As have their children.

Resistance must be assertive (assertive means being nice, but firm. Repeat: Nice, but firm).

Showing that you fear his reactions when you comment on his drinking guide him to do what you've just let him know will shut you up!

I know that there are reasons you give in; some of them are good reasons. But giving in is not the answer. Giving in won't change the danger; it surely won't change him. It won't make him nice so he'll never mention it again, especially all the way home.

Assertiveness is taught, not thought up. The lucky girls got that teaching since they were toddlers; you probably didn't. A licensed counselor, in two or three sessions, can teach you the simple (but not always easy) skills of assertiveness—being nice, but firm. Tell her that is your sole reason for seeing her—coaching on assertiveness skills. Invest time in two or three books from the library on assertiveness; scan and them all. Practice. You are quite smart so you'll get this fairly simple trick in no time at all. Your main block is believing that it's not nice to be honest or to state your wishes or needs. You know what to do about that! (Whatever it takes.)

> **Psych Note**: Sadly, animals who develop Learned Helplessness never go back to being themselves afterward. They continue in that state. They may recover slightly, but they never return to their original "personality."
>
> Researchers turned up the level of electric shocks to where they were even more painful, but the dogs just lay there; they still made no further efforts to be free. Worse, when researchers opened the doors to their cages, the animals stayed where they were. They had to be dragged out of the cages.
>
> Your physician, your minister, Alanon, your Yellow Pages: All offer forms of help to overcome what happens to the spirit that has been bullied, put down, emotionally abused. Help is out there. If you are stuck, despite the availability of help, then look at yourself to see if you've fallen into Learned Helplessness. If so, you need a counselor who is experienced in working with abused (physically or verbally) women.
>
> The Good News is that, while animals never recover well, people can and do.
>
> I call it "Learned Recovery." It requires outside intervention though because getting through closed mental doors is comparable to trying to be your own dentist. An outsider is needed.
>
> Find the right female counselor to take your hand, so to speak, and gently lead you back, out of the cage of erroneous learning.

The Way Home

Talk to your primary care physician about your situation, and be open about your level of stress—as well as your desire to not use medication unless both you and your doctor understand the medication is not a cure. Often changes in diet, or increases in exercise, and other lifestyle changes are sufficient to bring you relief. But you must remember that there's no complete cure without the inner work. And that this is almost impossible alone.

I do recommend short-term counseling—preferably from a licensed female counselor who has a great deal of experience in dealing with abused women. (I stress your need for a female counselor because I've seen a number of cases where a woman in pain fell into becoming enamored of her kind, understanding man, sensitive and helpful, a listener and guide. This event closes several doors that need to stay open for healing.)

(Note: I've never met a drinker's woman who hadn't been verbally and-or emotionally abused. It's what the alcohol does to the man's brain that produces this behavior.)

Some of you may find that you need medication long-term. This is particularly true for women in, near, or beyond menopausal age. The tragic reality is that enough stress creates physical and mental conditions that may never completely be healed. Menopause brings changes that seem to increase this possibility. In any case, just as you would work toward building strength to get out of a wheelchair, focus on building and rebuilding yourself. Believe me, you definitely have the resources and the equipment to do so—once the pressure lets up a little. I have never seen a spunkier group of women!

Another Important Consideration

If separation is in your best interest, then it's extremely important that, before you get into another relationship, you learn all you can about the twists to your personality. Not evil or crazy, not broken, just bent, and they will continue to cause you trouble until you unwind them. Learn all you can about the way you choose a partner. Talk to friends about all this. What initially attracts you to someone? What about a guy causes you to perk up? List some of those things here; learn more about yourself. (She's cool. And spunky.)

1. _____

2. _____

3. _____

Having thoughts of finding a great guy in the future is normal—but avoid dwelling on it just for now. Here's why: Those good-feeling fantasies lead to being blinded to things you need to watch out for in any new interest. You also must have time and help to heal a bit while you reprogram your "picker," which very likely is a bit off-kilter. You can have friendships; just guard against romanticizing—for now.

List on the next page at least three qualities you want to watch for and run when you see them in any new prospect for romance.

1. _____

2. _____

3. _____

Let's go over again some other reasons to stay detached emotionally for a while:

- You will still be attracted to the same type of person as your last partner.
- You will still behave the same way once you are attracted—if he misbehaves even slightly, and likely in a way that can invite a bully, being all apologetic for speaking your truth.
- You will still tend to overlook signs that this man is a lot like the last one—and resist the truth, that if so, this relationship will turn out like the last one.
- You will still hang on for dear life, even in the face of ominous signs, because of your mistaken ideas of romantic love.

It's like entering a critical care unit. Before resuming life as usual, wait until healing is established. You need to explore what attracts you in a man, and why, explore attraction to an entirely different personality or look, and staying alert for any signs that this man may be more like the last one than you wish. Explore your innermost reasons for hanging into a relationship long after other women would bail, and a few other things.

You can do these things very well in a group—a co-dependent group or Alanon, or a therapy group.

Unless you make a few small alterations in your picker's , you'll likely be attracted to the same kind of personality. The type of men you are attracted to resides in a template installed when you were just a very little girl. The snag could have crept in anywhere between then and now too, so take your time in investigating these things about yourself.

Worse, if you get entangled too soon, you probably still won't have the skills you need to stop trouble should it begin.

In fact, it is possible to create a bully. This can happen if you are continually bowing to his every whim. This usually occurs because you are attentive and caring—and don't want to be rejected.

Getting into another romance before you gain new skills will almost surely to get into another relationship just like the last. Countless women have done just that. Probably most drinkers's women. Probably some you know.

Some have done it two, three, and more times. Some ten! Oh, yeah, I'm telling the truth.

The cure? Well, for starters . . .

1. Self-research (with help—books, friends/counselors). Ask for their input on your choice of men and your way of conducting a relationship. Do not speak! Just listen—and write every bit of their answers down.

2. Learning (reading, or from others) which of your traits may need tweaking.

3. Get help deciding on which ONE to work on first. (Only one at a time to avoid a crash.)

4. Learn new ways and tricks to experiment with and practice the good ones as often as you can.

5. Stay grateful for every opportunity to pull out one of your new tricks again for practice—don't fear those times.

Your natural loving, forgiving, and compassionate self wants to believe the best of a potential partner, especially if he's cute and funny—and maybe has a good job. At this point, you'll want to think that he will not harm you. But that same unproven, untried trust has cost millions of women their lives— whether because emotionally damaged or actual death.

You don't have to be with a violent man to die from your relationship, as you see in looking at what you've learned about stress.

And at the first, tiniest signal that he can be ugly—to anyone—back off. Slow down. Step off the train. Cut bait!

The longer you put it off (especially for fear you're doing the wrong thing), the harder it is to do.

Spend yourself lavishly on people who love and appreciate you, people who are considerate of you and good to you.

Strictly avoid people who either look down on you, or put you down in any way, or who bully you, or attempt to control you—especially by making you feel bad about yourself.

Another thing: Holding back your emotions of "falling in love" will make you sensitive to those early warnings of trouble—you know, the things you've said, "I should have known better—I saw him do such and such early on, but I ignored it."

The reason you didn't "see" was that your mind was clouded with a fantasy of love. Just as if you were starved, you would to fall upon a hamburger, so can your emotional starvation cause you to leap upon a new, untried, prospect.

(Note: The experts estimate that it takes about 10,000 practice hours to become a master concert pianist, or a Rembrandt-quality artist. But all you need is a fairly comfortable assertiveness skill—which means the ability to be firm while being nice. And you get it only by practicing it. The lucky girls learned it from those around them, and have practiced it all their lives; that's why the do it so well. Not because they are better than you in any way!)

If you don't quite make your 10,000 hours, even half way means you'll still be a champion of the skill. If you practice any one of these tricks only *once*, you're still one notch better at it than you were.

The point: Practice!

Think about doing any one of these tricks and mark down that thinking as one practice. You think you're cheating? Nope. Your subconscious can't tell the difference between your fantasy and your real action; it responds the same to both. Simply thinking about doing the trick carries sticking power.

Those of you who are like me, who love to make checkmarks on a tally sheet when you've been a good girl (or stick a gold star on) can speed up the process of learning that way too. Make yourself a tally sheet or chart. Just write the name of the trick with blank space under to put the stars.

Hey, Did a Magic Want Just Wave And Make It Possible to be Perfect?

At first, your new ways escape you in the heat of the moment. That's to be expected. The old ways are reflex, simple habits. When you tense up, you can go into a minor brain freeze. Your new ways can desert you for the time being. Fortunately, the remedy is simple:

As soon as you realize you've jammed up, plug in one of your new tricks. The best one is probably Stretch 'Em and Move Along; they are practically fail-safe, in practically every tense situation. (Especially when they are enhanced with Air Talk, like, "Oh, is that smoke I smell?")

Here's how we know that you naturally have the traits, qualities, skills, and inner beauty that make you a valuable human being: You could never have become a drinker's woman without being all those qualities.

* * *

MASTERY

Pull out one or two points from this chapter that you want to absorb totally or fast, and write them here.

1. _____

_____

2. _____

_____

Chapter 9

Are You Safe?
(and a discussion of "It Can't Happen to Me")

> **SECOND NOTICE**
>
> Domestic violence is common
> in the homes of over-drinkers!
>
> If your drinker has ever been violent,
> once he's had even a small amount to drink,
> you may not be safe.

The reason so many women say, "It can't happen to me?"
It's because the idea that he will hurt-scar-kill you is so scary that it raises near the highest anxiety you are capable of. We've discussed how uncomfortable that level of anxious arousal is terribly uncomfortable—every nerve in your body is pushing on every muscle (which is what "tension" is—and your subconscious knows you need to shut it down or you'll be useless—or shatter.

And your subconscious remembers it has that handy built-in black hole where it can dump uncomfortable thoughts.

The reason you flood out the idea that you may not be safe from him and shove it into the black hole (where nothing can escape) is that you cannot deal with the idea that you may be seriously harmed by him.

Let's slow this down. Take a deep breath. Okay, let's proceed.

A substantial number of women who have been killed by their partner have told families and friends, "Oh, no, he wouldn't do that!"

The horrendous anxiety such an idea produces. And what it represents: perhaps the need to pull up stakes and scram, financial hardship, losing a good neighborhood or school? happens when you get an overload of anxiety?

Of my personal acquaintances who have been killed by their partner, both of their bodies were found by their children. Right! Brain Freeze, sweep the dark closet clean.

Breathe.

Let's just look at the facts.

The overblown (abnormal) jealousy and explosive rage result from brain changes due to damage. Join those serious emotional problems to the damage being done in the drinker's judgement and behavior control brain areas and the result will be very high incidence of domestic violence.

Damage to his behavior control brain area and also to his judgement-decision center join this sometimes fatal mix.

His rapidly accelerating emotional responses are due to his gradual loss of brain cells in the areas of controlling his emotions, his behavior, and very poor judgement—again due to cell damage and death in the frontal brain. At any moment he can become enraged and explode into violence.

This is difficult for some women to accept, even though they have observed him exploding in a temper more than once. A woman may frequently question his love for her. yet shut out the mental idea, the possibility—thus, never preparing for it, never planning what to do if threatened, never having an escape plan. *Do you have an escape plan?*

Any woman whose partner is or ever has been violent must construct an escape plan—perhaps even practice it, if only mentally. It's fairly simple, and very easy to put together—this escape plan.

So why do almost none of the most threatened women create one?

Because they are still fixated on who he used to be. Perhaps that guy couldn't harm them—but the guy in "today's picture" may be more able.

Seeing him as the wonderful guy she fell for, if only in his heart, and (importantly) believing that if she just does the right things he won't get upset and she won't get hurt.

You see what she's done?

She's made it all into something under her control.

But violence is not under the control of the victim or the intended victim. Where did she get such an idea?

From his saying, "Well, if you hadn't said-done so and so, I wouldn't have blown up. You brought this on yourself." And she's heard it every time he has crossed the line. "I only do bad because you're imperfect. You see? I'm not bad, it's you who gets it started!"

He may even add, without thinking, "You know how I get!" As if knowing he's a violent horse's butt should protect her. Well, does it? Has it?

I doubt it.

These women (thousands and thousands of them) pour themselves into fixing themselves, working on all the things in them and their surroundings that could trigger him. Eventually she will hardly ever speak because she's found so many things she says get him riled. She will suffer terrible anxiety, until it slips into being severe depression. (Remember Learned Helplessness?) And some of them, after a bit longer, will not step out of the cage, even if the door is open and all their needs are provided. They are full of fear, but mostly they are shut down.

Early on, they beat themselves when they say or do something that he says upsets him. At some point, they agree that they are getting what they deserve.

Most have ignored the bad stuff and kept him in the Prince outfit. Believing that's who he really is—inside.

What have I said before? Oh, yes—"Hitting is not love," and blaming your victim for your own bad behavior is not love. Baby, what if he's already beyond the ability to turn back into the Prince. For more than a day. (Most can fake it briefly, as you have likely already experienced.)

This chapter is extremely important for every woman with a man who drinks too much. It is important to women whose partners are violent even though they don't drink or use drugs. Our culture and movies and fairy tales have implanted ideas in us that simply aren't true. Fairy tales are—fairy tales.

The number of murders committed by men on their women are listed at 2,000 per year. All parties interested in this problem admit the number is vastly under-estimated. We discover that the 2,000 number is actually counting only the murders where there was enough proof to convict the killer.

That number covers only the killers against whom they had enough evidence, and that a jury (or just a judge) could clearly see that he was guilty. Remember that there likely are as many, walking around your town or close by, who got away with it because they couldn't prove anything.

All the experts say those numbers will continue to grow every year.

The numbers also tell us that an average of 40 women are killed in every state. Do you know how many in your state? It's probably right there on the Internet. Check it out.

Forty dead women in *your* state this year, young women usually, most mothers. One killed in our country every 9 days, on average.

And what are we doing about it?

A little, but not enough by a long shot.

It is my hope that the information I give you here will save your life.

Him

Alcohol dulls judgement, and then it dulls behavior control; this means that emotional outbreaks will immediately burst forth.

Some women say their man would never hurt them, but the guy who wouldn't hurt them—if he's still there at all—happens to be drunk. If a man is going to become violent, even for the first time, the odds say it will be when he takes a drink.

The brain is complicated and only a few of its functions are fully understood, so we can't explain why a man can drink so much that he passes out, and then, without warning rise up from that unconscious state like a maniac and kill.

Many, many women have thought their guy was asleep or passed out. As they began to gather things to leave, he came to in a drunken rage , attacked and kill her, often in front of her children, then he will have absolutely no memory of it later.

> What do most people say (or think) when a man kills his partner? They ask this: "What did **she** do?" (Unspoken: "to deserve it?") Most of us need to work on that too. The underlying idea goes deep in almost all cultures and societies.

This chapter comes to you in large part because I know that his rage, so scary to you that you blank it out (your own denial system), and it can fall on your children too. Think: The babies this victim I spoke of was holding.
And my own child.

Avoiding thinking about all of this is almost universal, your denial system wants you to believe it can't happen to you. To think otherwise is just too stressful, possibly overwhelming.

Compounding the danger: Alcohol dulls any love feelings, dulling those areas of the brain that love, and those that care about consequences.

When attacked, even threatened, you are most likely to go into Brain Freeze, meaning you will not be able to adequately protect yourself—or others.

A note in case for those who have already been hit: The chances that he will repeat this, do it again and worse, are practically 100 percent.
For a drinker, 200 percent.

Many men truly mean it when they say, "Never again, I swear to you!" but alcohol dulls all the machinery of holding back, of self-restraint, especially under emotional pressure. And he is quite capable of producing out of nothing powerful rages. For him to react, when unrestrained, in a way he has before must be expected. Beginning to think this way can save your life—or the life of a child, or save you from being crippled, or carrying facial scars from cuts or acid or worse for the rest of your life. This is serious business, but the fearful Inner Child in you doubts herself, her own judgement, and every day she spends being put down and criticized chops it down further.
I'm telling you that staying with a man who has already hit you, especially a man who over-drinks, or who uses certain drugs is one of the most dangerous men on earth to the woman who lives with him. This is the longest shot you could possibly bet gambling with your own survival.
Heroin addicts and heavy marijuana users are rarely violent. (Rumor is that weed gets into prisons via uniformed men who

use this method of sedating the herd to make them safer.) You have learned that, due to the brain changes (damage) inflicted by alcohol, brain parts that do not grow back, he's extremely unlikely to tur himself around, much less stay that way.

But here's my point: You have been sustained by this dream of him changing for so long, that dream in turn being sustained by every romance novel you read or chick flick you watch. In the face of this dream implanted in most little girls, reality doesn't have much of a chance—not until it gets soooo bad most people would have fled long ago. That dream, fantasy, can keep you in this destructive living condition until the stress and other afflictions of the over-drinker and your deteriorating life and lifestyle—until all of that breaks you for real. Your emotional health will give way first, and you'll become either over-emotional or numb: a zombie.

Next to go will be your mental health That's your loss of confidence in yourself and your thinking and decisions; it's anxiety that begins to spread into every moment of your life; it's depression that smothers you, keeps you tied down with no desire—or ability—to do better.

And, while every bit of these things were going on, the last bastion, your physical health will break down, seriously break down. You will have had physical problems which have worsened, and now they become life-threatening.

All because someone planted the dream that bad guys can turn good if only . . . .

And so—I wrote this book. And a stream of articles, all to begin educating women to the reality of relationships, partnerships, love. Success in any of these depends on a whole, healthy mind and emotional stability. With an over-drinking problem, he drops the ball in all relationship areas, but what makes it devastating is that you too are losing your capacity and abilities—from emotional damage and the physical-mental impact of stress.

All these things lead to arguments and bearing grudges and much anger toward each other.

And now I'm telling you that he may become dangerous.

In this chapter I'm opening myself to you—to the world, actually—to share, not only my experiences working with and for with many women who have been battered, and not only from the research I do keeping up with the latest information on the problem, but I share just a tad of my own experiences. That is scary; people react to my history in different ways. I have no way of knowing how you react to this type of discussion, and I have no way to help you digest it. I will tell you that it's perfectly acceptable for you to need a break.

I don't want to turn any of you away from things some of you need to look at. Promise me now that, if some of my "stuff" unsettles you, that you will just skip over that part, and go on to read the things beyond that point. Not all of you, but some of you need to know where I am coming from as I write this chapter.)other things I believe you need to know.

*I remember--the first time he hit me. I went into shock. I had just turned 15, and had dated him since I was 13 and he had never hit me; he knew one of the reasons I ran away from home with him three weeks after my 15th birthday was because my father beat me. All I could think was, "How could he **do** this?" I couldn't believe it. But soon, he was falling all over me, petting me and telling me how sorry he was, and that he would never do it again.*

He did. (And he said that many of those times over the years.)

Some people have such painful memories left from their experiences that reading mine may set off their anxiety. No one should ever be forced to deal with their own emotional scars; not even encouraged to until they are strong enough. It is desirable to "deal" with them because "dealing with them" is part of the process of breaking free.

(I pray that you are now in a place where the batterer cannot hurt you, ever again.)

"Dealing with" the after-effects of abuse can be difficult. You will do it faster and with less pain if you consult a licensed therapist. If money is a problem, be up-front with her and offer to pay her a little every other week, or between sessions with you coming back once the last session is paid. I wish we professionals could do all of our work for free, but the world isn't yet enlightened sufficiently. (Doctors too.) The work you will do as you examine yourself and your experiences with reliable guidance may sometimes an ordeal, but it will be well worth every step.

Take your time. No one gets a gold medal in this work

I will tell you that writing about these parts (plural) of my life (and yes, I left one batterer for another—an outcome I've mentioned as a possibility for your future unless you do the work to heal yourself.

Some of my past is still painful, like the shattering of my nest—that had my babies in it. I had five children (three by the time I was 18). Pain like when my husband came in and put the dead body of my baby in my arms. It's been almost 50 years, but it's still there.

It is scary to share this experience, I rarely can predict others's reactions to it. Remembering still brings pain, although my own work on "dealing with it" has made it bearable. Most of the time. Not always on his birthday. Or the anniversary of the day he died. Every few years I seem to fall apart on one of those days. In my own healing, I learned that my pain was normal, and I shouldn't let it or other people intimidate me over it. When I hurt, it's okay to cry.

Just so is it for you.

* * *

An over-drinker's rage and jealousy are so much a part of drinking disorders that they have separate names in psych text books: "alcoholic rage" and "alcoholic jealousy." These forms of jealousy and rage are in a class by themselves, due to the alcohol-induced brain changes that create them.

As he deteriorates, he sits on an unstable reservoir of explosive inner he's angry. His life is steadily getting worse, his relationships, his finances, his family, and no one understands him! At least that's his take on it.

All these troubles give him a full supply of irritants to be angry about. The rage born of his muddled thinking and determination to blame the world rather than himself, creates an ever-bubbling cauldron.

And an over-drinker's jealousy can be triggered by the slightest event—or none: another man smiling at his woman, or looking at her, or not looking but he thinks the guy is looking, or he thinks her eyes are aimed in the direction of a passing man, or some other hare-brained pipe dream he spits out in a split-second. His ideas do not have to make sense for him to feed on them. He has come to savor his rage, it's his proof that the world is out to get poor innocent him. And all those thoughts feel good to him.

Eventually his rages easily escape his control.

The circulating chemicals and the damaged brain centers eventually run the show, not an intelligent mind. And this occurs much earlier than most people want to believe. I put it at the time he crosses into the Third Stage in Chapter 5.

His emotional arousal and the energy it produces coupled with his anger and loss of behavior control are what make him dangerous.

In an instant, overwhelming rage can explode in him at minor events, or nothing at all. He will have interpreted the event as a threat—to his ego, his manhood, his ability to drink. He comes to rage inside (most of the time) at the rest of the world, at himself, at the life he has created for himself but blames others for.

And who is usually nearby—most accessible, available for fielding his blast, either aimed at her or the stress of exploding at something else in her presence. Who absorbs the products of his inner rage?

Right. His woman.

You.

He can come to be a splashing can of gasoline, its fumes drifting around, waiting for the tiniest spark.

You can want so much for him to go back to being the nice guy that you tend to minimize his numerous explosions and the harms they cause in your mental and emotional wellbeing. And the more precarious things get, the greater your fear that something will shatter your world.

A part of you is fighting against awareness that your nest may be falling apart. You may say that it only happens when he's angry, and that if you "straighten up" it won't happen so often.

(Sometimes I think women do this because it enables them to feel like they have some control.)

For some, the fear of a shattered nest is great because you don't trust yourself to be able to make it financially without him.

Hm-m, what could the rapid cure for that be?

Consult with the women at your local women's shelter for an answer.

Another thing that will help greatly: Your "today picture."

Most women fear how they can make it without him. At first it's difficult, as any huge adjustment is, and if you have children, financial difficulties may be problems for some time. But so would hospital bills be a problem for some time.\

Maybe a break isn't as hard as you think.

If you're savvy enough to read this book for answers, you have more than enough brain and moxie to make it. Drinkers's women have been beaten down terribly. The worse their drinker got, the more he needed to feel superior and—well, you were there, convenient.

Many of you have been robbed of your self-confidence, but my vast experience with this problem has shown that not only are almost every one of you some of the strongest, smartest, kindest, most capable people in the world. And many of you believe you've lost it, but you're also quick, and bright, and spunky!

You haven't lost it. I've discovered that the spunky gal you really are has just gone into hiding. It doesn't take much to get her back out and lending a helping hand to your progress.

I find masses of spunk in drinkers's women; it has been in hiding, waiting for someone to dig it out.

Now, if you fear you won't be able to cope, align yourself as fast as possible with a group of women. Let them work with you, to heal, to rebuild. It *will* come.

There's a saying in Alcoholics Anonymous, something about healing, like sometimes it comes quickly, sometimes slowly, but it *always* comes when you begin to work on it.

I have no statistics on this but it's a reality: I have never seen or heard of a woman who broke free from a nasty relationship committing suicide. But I *have* seen and heard of many who did not make the break do so.

So far gone and filled with self-dislike, she does harm to herself, vents her rage and pain on herself, not the one who has set it all up. She hurts herself because someone else has hurt her. It just doesn't make sense to do that, does it?

Do not waste all that you are and will be learning; you soon can help countless others.

* * *

Dynamics of Anger that Becomes Rage

If he doesn't dump his rage it builds, swelling, pushing closer and closer to the surface, and then it explodes—molten lava from his inner hell. Stop and think now: A sane person doesn't react with an explosion of rage and blaming to an event the size of a mosquito, or one of any size, come to think of it.

All you need to do to guarantee that more terrible things will happen is add alcohol to this endlessly failing recipe.

You can become so depressed that you begin to think your safety isn't important. This is an explanation that comes easy to you—so think about how sad that is!

Oh, yes, my darling, you have a mix of skills and talents and traits that no one else on earth has, and God didn't make a mistake when He created you and wired you up. After all the work of creation, of filling you with knowledge, all the suffering you can now make have meaning when you help others, what a waste if you even get injured, much less killed. And you are the only one who can make that happen. You will have to enlist others, but it is only you who can take that first step.

Some of you think, as I did, "Well, maybe he's not that bad. Maybe it really is me." If you reach this state, it is sufficient proof that he already is "that bad." Only someone "that bad" could inflict such personal harm on someone they sometimes profess to love. This is a mind that is coming unwrapped, and nothing but his taking a first step into some form of help can stop the unravelling of that mind. It will continue so long as he drinks alcohol.

One guideline for monitoring your safety is staying alert to the possibility, at any time, that he may carry that continuously boiling inner state, and that at any time his fragile control over how he responds to anything upsetting is down. You pay attention to and continually assess his potential loss of control.

Mind you, his rages aren't about what he says they are! It's not bad drivers, coworkers, authority figures, bosses and politicians, a burnt steak, or you. His rages are the result of unrelenting inner mental and emotional pressure coming his own backed-up fight or flight chemicals and lack of sufficient personal control. Analyzing the situation, you see that of his choices with that backed-up chemistry, Flight or Fight, he is not likely to "fly" except to a bar. If he chooses that, do not interfere.

If he doesn't choose that, suggest it. Go to the refrigerator and pop the top on a beer. While it is more alcohol on top of too much, the gesture has great surprise value. His tendency is that, instead of seeing you as the enemy, to see you as his best friend.

Without some form of intervention at these times, either your being able to Move Along, or being able to get him a drink to buy you time until you can Move Along, he is sure to latch onto anything that happens that he thinks justifies dumping his raging chemistry. Mean words, blame, raging, hitting.

That's because he stays at a level of easy ignition.

Normal anger is an emotion meant to energize us to make changes—but his has become all twisted up. He remembers, if only subconsciously, that he feels better after he blows (because he's burning off those uncomfortable rage chemicals).

He also erroneously believes his rage is a way to maintain control over things—everything. You. It's his way to get others to do what he wants them to. Subconsciously he seeks events that can become excuses for blowing up.

> **Psych Note:** Subconscious means he isn't consciously aware of this process. The involvement of his subconscious in his raging connects to whatever he blames for that anger, and also remembers how rewarding blasting it all out is. These subconscious processes makes it impossible to reason with him. Reasoning requires conscious thought. In most cases, the subconscious is far stronger than the conscious mind.

When you sense any tension in a man who has already hit you, Move Along. Smell smoke, have to go to the bathroom. You must save yourself. One thing is that you **do not disagree with him.**

Do not try to reason with him.

When he is mentally and emotionally in this state, disagreement on *anything* is a spark—it's the lit match.

It can be totally unrelated to what is being discussed in the argument, but when it aggravates him, all that chemistry of rage now bursts through the new outlet.

Trying to reason with him gives him a bunch of new things to argue against. Avoid arguing; don't try to justify yourself; be quiet as possible. Sometimes pretending fear is enough to feed their ego, but then again, I've seen it fire up their God-complex and fuel more rampage.

The only way you can win (survive mentally, emotionally, and perhaps physically) in these situations is to agree with him.

At least appear to agree with whatever he's saying.

Disagreement, or him sensing your disagreement when he is all wound up, is playing Russian Roulette with his fists (or worse).

You do not lose face for backing down. You aren't on PBS News. What's more, he likely won't remember much of the debacle later.

And you do NOT need to protect your ego now, no matter what he says—unless he says he's beating you for doing that thing.

A violent man doesn't get better so long as he takes even one drink; he only gets worse.

Agree with a man who even possibly can become violent.

Your Inner Actress is most certainly capable of playing the part of a caring friend who generally agrees with whatever he's ranting about.

Emblazon on your mind that when you try to reason with rage, he is ready now for war and he can interpret anything you say as fighting against him. Then you become a justifiable target (in his warped judgement). Do not try to reason beyond the first attempt. If it fails, don't throw rosemary on it. Move Along, girl!

You can be sure he will not change the thinking that sets off his rage now, no matter what you say or do. But he *will* find something in whatever you say or do to use as an excuse for exploding on you.

No one on earth can bring him to his senses when he's at the point of rage. Especially not you. That's partially because he's too accustomed to you being his garbage dump. Don't even try it. Later you might be able to express your thoughts on the subject.

In responding to him, timing your actions is how to control what happens. You know that anything you say or do with any appearance of disagreement is the spark he's waiting for, an excuse to blow up!

But doing something nice, something unexpected, like saying convincingly, "I could use a cold beer right now. How 'bout you?" That or something like it will produce a Brain Freeze (no matter how small). Carry through by getting beer and handing it to him and appearing to be drinking one too (or really drink it). You have now opened a good space to Move Along.

You are not backing down; you are side-stepping.
When you go into silent of backing-off mode, you are not backing off. You are stopping a steam roller that is capable of mowing your grass.

Understand that such worries are ego-based, those are the things he thinks are important, but not you. And his opinion of you cannot be helped in any way by making a point in an argument. Clam up! Clamp 'Em.

How often has getting the last word worked for you anyway?

His nasty comments may only be bait now, doing what usually riles you up—for what? To do whatever he wants. So just let him. Do not ever bring up a contentious topic when he's drinking. Save it. Save it for when?

Right! Save it for the hangover.
Beware taking his bait.
Agree with him. "Yes, Honey."

He is capable of saying anything to get you riled, not because it's true, but because it opens up a path to release his tension. "I only blow up like this at you because you fight me on *everything*. You know I'm going to get angry! But you do it anyway! You deserve what you get!" and so on.

He' sometimes adds, "You're crazy-stupid,-sick," whatever hurtful thing comes to mind. All of that is merely to taunt you—he's not saying it because it's true. To taunt you into arguing back at him.

Whatever he says you have done to "make" him angry, let it go with a show of agreeing.

I haven't found another technique for handling a man who can be violent, Surprise! Brain Freeze! Move Along.

As to really blaming yourself, have you noticed that even when you comply with his wishes, he can stay angry? Come up with something else to rant about? I bring it up just to demonstrate the silliness of most of what he's saying.

Anger

Anger is a dangerous emotion for anyone, especially a male. Research shows that testosterone levels are powerful predictors of a man's level of rage (and of violent behavior).

Anger is especially dangerous in a male with an impaired brain—and a drinker's brain is definitely impaired—in all the important places.

Alcohol steadily lowers his testosterone levels, but it takes a long time, likely years for it to diminish his tendency to rage.

> **Psych Note:** His steadily shrinking testosterone levels are why he has trouble getting and keeping an erection, why he needs more and more stimulation to become aroused, why he demands that you do something you'd rather not to "get him off."
>
> You *and* he need to know that alcohol actually causes his penis and testicles to steadily shrink.
>
> I am convinced that if this news ever makes it out (most avenues are financed by companies with interests in selling alcohol) men wouldn't be as eager to belly up to the bar.

His ever-bubbling cauldron of rage builds primarily because of his increasing frustration over his out-of-control life. It isn't you.

You see his control slipping in other ways too: He pukes on himself or in places he knows he should not. He pees the bed—or worse. He wobbles and staggers, stumbles, and falls, speaks insanity with words hard to understand because of slurring. All of these are signs of his brain's loss of control. He cannot control his speaking, walking, or his bladder. Nor his mouth or rage.

And yet he accuses you of being insane.

His rages are terrifying because they can explode without warning, and because they can escalate out of his control (and yours too). As to trying to control his rage, realize that there's nothing, *nothing* you can say or do once the pin pricks the balloon. At that point, no one can change what happens next. Nor is there anything you can say that can reliably slow him down, much less stop him (short of heavy drugs and weapons).

The point is this: Stop trying to control his rage!

When you see any sign of it, Move Along.

The uncomfortable, threatening, surprise factor associated with his rage increase a sense of danger to you. Gradually, this sense of danger is present so often that you can come to stay in a state of either readiness (anxiety) or giving up (depression, Learned Helplessness). Even when you're not around him.

Anxiety? When he's not around, you stay attentive to anything that might displease him. It becomes a constant part of your thinking. Whew! Aren't you tired? Do you know how much stress that adds to your load?

Don't allow anyone to label you as mentally disturbed. You are reacting exactly the way any other sane human would react to the same very unpleasant situation, where awful things can arrive by surprise. What living like this does to you or has done to you is not make you crazy; you have responded normally!

You react like any other sane person under the same stress, dealing with the same stress-ors.

Psych Note: The definition of "anxiety" is a form of fear without a rational cause!

Pul-leeze! Your watchfulness for anything that can bring on his rage is not nuts, and it's definitely not anxiety! Anxiety is a state of fear when no threat exists.

Anti-anxiety medication can somewhat relieve the *discomfort* of ongoing dread, but it is not a cure.

The cure? Either he changes, or you move out from his influence.

If you burn your hand on the stove, you don't relieve it by taking medicine, but by taking your hand off the burner.

No form of stress can improve so long as the stress-or still exerts pressure.

When he blows, the over-drinker's inflated denial system is immediate and so-so slick. He instantly blames his emotional responses and behaviors on some external cause—never on the truth, which is his own increasing inability to think clearly or control his emotions or behavior or life.

To him, his rage is always justified. He has no concern for the very real mental and emotional harm his own behavior wreaks on others. He will go to just about any length to establish his innocence and others's culpability.

Arguing about whether he's right is useless. It's not only useless, but at some point it becomes dangerous—and that danger is present from its first moment if he's had anything to drink at all in the last hour or so.

Your best bet is "Yes Honey," and a slow, gentle Move Along with air talk expressing a possible emergency—smoke! bathroom break! someone knocking at the door!

Defending yourself from his verbal attacks is wasted spirit, wasted because it simply will not work—cannot work. For him to understand your side requires a fully functioning brain. He is losing, or has lost his.

What protesting or defending yourself, or arguing, are guaranteed to do, however, is stoke his inner fire. And now, if it wasn't already, it will instantly be fully directed toward you!

Do not argue with whatever he says is the cause of his rage! If you must respond, show empathy. And Move Along.

Your best (and safest) response is silence. Next to that, agreement. Sounds like this: "Yeah, you may be right."

This one response to almost anything he can spout can save your life.

* * *

A Thought

Go figure—when a man cheats, his woman almost always thinks first about doing harm to the woman involved!

It's as if we believe getting rid of that particular woman will cure this cheating man.

As if getting rid of this one can fix whatever is making him cheat.

Wrong!

Even if you wiped out all of them (because cheating is almost never a one-time behavior), there's always a little girl somewhere just entering puberty whom he will soon consider fair game.

Although the cheating partner is in the wrong, this is true only if she knows he's committed. Likely he has told her that he is on the brink of separating or divorce, and she believes him.

The cheating problem lies solely in the cheater. That woman made no promises of fidelity to you. What's more she believes his stories of how awful his woman is and how he needs a little loving.

A cheating man is not the result of some flaw in his woman, as he tells the world. It is *his* interest, *his* willingness to wander, giving *himself* the permission to wander—those are the problem.

Cheating can be a form of addiction too, meaning you don't have much hope of changing that streak in him once it comes out.

I was raised in a very strict form of Baptist belief. The understandings gleaned from the Bible by these readers is that the man is the Master, the woman must bow to his wishes. All his wishes. I disliked this lifestyle, but didn't speak it. I no longer believe that a woman is to be treated as a slave. I heard more than once, when going for help to a minister, "Yes, I know it's a burden, but it's woman's penalty for tasting the apple and getting her husband to fall too."

(That attitude and those teachings almost kept me from ever finding sobriety, healing. I had a heck of a time overcoming my resentment.) My drinking and drug use began as a way to cope with the death of my baby, beaten by his father, and dying a few hours later from brain injury. The father had interrupted a beating of me to snatch up the baby, who was crying, and storm out of the tin trailer we lived in and head for the woods.

About 20 minutes later he returned holding out the limp body of my child to me. Ah, that's enough for now.

After years of doing what my religion demanded, staying with him, taking the beatings, the mistreatment, here's what happened. My grandmother, often distraught seeing the signs of beatings on me, bruises, black eyes, busted lips, sat me down one day to discuss getting away from that man.

She was a strict Baptist, a Sunday School teacher (for 75 years when she died at 88), but she was telling me I needed to get a divorce. I was in shock at her words. I had all my 16 years believed and lived by what preachers had taught me. The man is master; my duty under God is to take it and continue to be the best wife in the world.

Grandmother told me that day that her father (alcoholic) had beaten her mother and she had seen and hard it all through her childhood. When she was 16, her mother died a few days after a beating.

Then she told me that I must get away from this man. I responded by telling her that the Bible said we couldn't divorce. Then she said two things:

One: "No, you're wrong. I know some preachers preach that Jesus said we couldn't divorce, but that's not what he said. He said you couldn't remarry after divorce."

And Two: "You are allowed to divorce for cause of adultery—and you've told me you suspect that. But this man killed your child, and he has almost killed you, and surely God sees murder as serious a sin as adultery. Becky (that's what she called me), you must get away from this man. I will help you any way I can."

After about two weeks and another serious beating, I went to her for help. We made a plan, she financed my journey out of the area. He had threatened to kill me if I tried to leave him, and she wanted me to be far away.

I escaped. I divorced. I grieved, and at 16, with only a ninth grade education, I worked at whatever I could find to support myself.

And I began to drink. A lot.

It was my blessed escape from pain and fear and guilt—my fear of God alternating with rage at Him.

In any business contract, if either party breaks any term of that contract, the other party has the right to terminate the entire contract. I came to understand that a man who cheats on his wife is breaking his contract (his vows). He broke the bond, the contract, not the wife who left because of it.

He is dishonest, and a liar. He is an adulterer. That makes him is a contract-breaker.

And that broken contract set me free!

I tell you this story for those of you who have been given similar ideas about marriage. You are not the one breaking your contract; the strictest religions allow that divorce is allowed is there is "adultery."

He has already broken the contract. A broken contract is null and void.

Yes, I know. I haven't shared the horror of my child's death with you before. It is a difficult event for others to deal with, I watch them go into a kind of shock and I don't talk about it often out of consideration for others. And because, some 57 years later, it still hurts and I'm shedding tears as I write this.

I want you to know that I know our topic more than what I learned in my training, those six years of college majoring in psychology, and some 40 years of practice. I believe it's important to tell you some of my own experience. Many of you struggle with similar issues, and I pray they are not as harsh as mine though I know some of you have and have had it worse.

For those of you who have not been brutalized, thank your God and I do too. You may think that this chapter doesn't apply to you because you have not been through what others have. But you picked this book (with this title) for a reason, and you have received a lot of information on the man who drinks too much.

Even if you never need this information, every woman knows a woman who has or is living with a partner who over-drinks. You may know some who are being hit, although they are even more withdrawn than drinkers's women. And they are more committed to hiding their problem. Nevertheless, you now have the information you need to help her.

Vital Points in This Chapter

--1. Emotions work at near light speed; once burst out, his emotions and moods have little or no braking power.

--2. When not vented or tempered, emotions build up, creating a pressurized jam; they push for release.

--3. Built-up emotions are always on the edge of bursting through—at high power and without warning.

4. They *will* burst through at the first opening.

The Lay-Low Trick

1. Pay little attention to the things he says, don't take them to heart, don't react as if he speaks God's truth. He's only using you as an excuse to discharge his own pressure.

2. Whatever negative things he says, it's almost certainly not real in the sense he wants it to seem. Remember that just bait he throws out, trying to get you to argue--so he can use you as an excuse to explode. Then he can leave and go drink.

3. Stay alert for his signs of upset. You're already good at this; just step it up when drinking. Upon detecting any sign or anger, immediately CLAMP 'EM! Move Along!!

DO NOT STRETCH THE LIPS!!

He may take it dangerously wrong!

Clamp Lips and Jaws and Move Along.

You can only carry out the following "suggestions" to the best of your ability at the moment they are needed. We don't call them tricks because at moments of great upset and great danger you cannot count on reacting perfectly—and what is called for can vary greatly.

These suggestions are meant to be internalized. That way, they will at least be available if needed.

Slow down to read the following "suggestions." Take the few seconds to imagine yourself in the scene.

Imagine yourself acting out each step.

Do this as often as it comes to mind, imprinting them, making them more and more likely to pop up when you need them, despite your emotional state at the time.

However, you must understand that *nothing* can *assure* you will be safe at any time from a man who has already shown *any* violence toward you.

If he has hit you, you're mistaken to believe he won't go so far as to shoot you. It happens every few days.

Or that he wouldn't be capable of beating you to death. Or strangling you. Or knifing you. Or burning you. It happens every few days.

When I say "if he has ever hit you," it's the best marker I know at the moment to suggest that a man is capable of extreme violence. (The killing I spoke of earlier, you know, the young woman holding her two baby girls and him shooting all three of them to death—investigation concluded that he had hit her in the past, but it had been some time ago.

You will never know for sure. That is the whole reason I strongly advise going where you're safe.

Let's page down so the seven suggestions are all on the same page.

Seven Suggestions

1. **Exert effort to appear calm.** The way you look, your voice, what you say, how you move.

2. **Make him feel respected** and don't antagonize him. (Getting your points across can be done later when he is more sane. And safe.)

3. b. **Act calm.** He will feed on your excitement and step up doing whatever he believes has just cowed you.

4. **Move calmly** (unless violence is imminent). Moving quickly can act as a trigger on the backed up rage he's sitting on.

5. **Expect him to keep up the rampage** as long as the target (you) is still nearby, or until his rage chemicals go dry. **Don't count on him calming down.**

6. **Stay alert!** Rage and violence can be predictable-- sometimes, *and* unpredictable at others. (Do you think women have just stayed in the chair at the table while he went digging for his gun? That shooting was predictable. But he isn't likely to do that; he will most likely come at you by surprise. Stay alert throughout the event, get distance between you, and stay away until you are sure he's burned through his rage. Or forever. (These alcoholic rages are horrendous but usually the chemistry-fuel is used up fast. Usually. This too is not always predictable.

    Some men will sit on their rage, keep building it up intentionally, even after you're out of sight. Many such men may follow you somewhere and shoot you there. And maybe the momma or papa or sister who is sheltering you.

Every woman should contact their local women's shelter—just to be in the know if anyone they ever run into needs it.
That also would guarantee that every woman is educated in

best practices when trying to deal with, or leave, a violent man.

Even a few mental practices of these seven suggestions can make the difference for you. (Remember that violence tends to escalate—until it completely burns out. But you cannot positively tell if he's used up the rage chemicals when he slows down, or is just getting refueled.

For those of you who have suffered a beating, expect the next one to be as bad or worse than the last.

This urge in a man to beat his woman increases in power every time it's used.

It's like drinking. Forcing himself to stop without help results in a buildup of stuffed-down desires for a drink, and this causes overdoing it when he starts up again.

What to Expect

You never know *what* to expect from a man who has ever been violent. Still, there are some pretty firm rules of psychology that have been known to predict some of it.

> **Psych Note:** When a vending machine doesn't give you what you push the button for, what do you do?
>
> You try harder, don't you! You push the button harder, and many more times. Some people begin to rage at the machine and physically attack it—hitting or kicking it. This seems to be a wired-in response to not getting what we expect. The same thing exists in animals. So you must expect it from him.
>
> That means if he says or does something to get your goat, and you don't respond that way this time, what will he do?
>
> Right! He'll try again. Harder. Repeatedly.
>
> If you understand this is wired-in behavior, you will expect it and not be broken by the assault.

If you don't give him the response you usually would, at first he'll try harder to throw you off balance. Be ready.

He'll try even harder to push your button for the kind of response he's looking for. And he's looking for anything he can then use to justify what he's already set to do.

You hold your tongue—not because he's right but because he's a keg of dynamite, looking to get you to light his fuse.

"Yes Honey" is your fallback—but you must say it

convincingly, never sarcastically. His broken mind is still looking for a crack in your wall to slam through the rest of his rage.

* * *

And after he kills you, his lawyer will describe him to the jury as having been partially insane—because of the stresses you put him, being crazy and all, constantly arguing everything he said—with illustrations of your various behaviors. The one time you threw a vase. The one time you hit him back.

Oh, yes, he can use all those accusations as a defense in court for killing you!

And he will likely get off lightly because of it. The court records are full of such unhappy endings.

VITALLY IMPORTANT

Rage that is starting to cool can be easily and instantly inflamed again. A cloud passing overhead. A gnat.

I've never known a man who stopped hitting his woman—and stayed stopped—unless he got sober in a very strict program and stayed sober. I hear it happens, but I have never seen it in 40 years. That would seem to indicate that such cases of "healing" and staying healed are rare indeed.

Oh, yes! Be advised: Once the former violent over-drinker drinks again, they will eventually also hit again.

Your situation is more demanding and complicated when you have children to care for and protect. Because of the confusion around them, their emotions will be jumbled, their own denial strong; to mentally survive the chaos they find themselves in they will tend to take sides.

Don't get too upset at them for whatever they say about the situation or you or your mate. You can help them now by overlooking what is surely only a psychological protection they have put up for themselves. You can ward off more harm to them by explaining why they don't need to take sides, but they are allowed if they want to. Let them see that you know they care about both of you. Let them see and hear that both of you are to blame.

Most mothers are wounded deeply when their children champion him and blame her. Right now, gird up your loins for just such attacks because it is the most common. Know why? They have heard you yell at him, etc. They see you under heavy stress, while he is absent and the childish mind takes that as absence of meanness. Be ready for that; it's young, immature minds coping best they can. They likely will change in time, especially if you keep telling it's both of your faults. They have heard what he says to and about you—and if he's an over-drinker, you can be sure he attributes all of the trouble to you.

They have seen and heard you when your last nerve is shattered and you scream at him and throw a cup. He's out drinking, so they see you—your depression, your anger, all of which is perfectly normal, but they don't get the full picture of their father's behavior.

Worse: If you try to tell them much of it, they'll back off. That's because they're again emotionally overloaded.

They are truly conflicted: After blaming you for yelling at him, they'll turn around and blame you for not standing up for yourself. (I've heard that story countless times.)

I tell you these depressing facts so that, if you face similar situations, you'll know that you aren't the worst parent in the world, that you aren't alone, the only mother that has been rejected as the demon.

The best you can do is refuse to be triggered into anger with them (which is so easy to fall into when you are hurt or depressed and they say hurtful things). They are hurt and confused and need to make sense of it. They take sides. With gusto.

Best you can, focus on protecting them—but don't let up on protecting yourself. Try not to argue—with them or him in their presence. Do a lot of Move Along.

Finding something fun to do is still a great prescription in these trying times.

If you fear the impact of separation on your children, weigh out your decision again. You may have to decide whether it is better that they be emotionally wounded now by separation than be crippled, disfigured, or dead—or coming in to find their mother that way, as has happened in many cases.

The Good News: The violent man won't likely hurt

children who think he's the hero!

* * *

To save themselves discomfort, people on the outside of your house can refuse to believe that you live in hell; it's easier for some of them (especially his friends and family) to believe you are the bad guy. This is almost as difficult as when your children take that stance.

Best for you is to drop your concern about what these people think for the time being. Perhaps in time, maybe years down the road, they will see things differently. It has, however, been my experience and my observation that people who react that way are rarely worth much effort to keep close.

Don't allow the opinions of your children (or other family members) to make you feel like the bad guy. And do not try to convert them to seeing you as a victim, not the bad guy—at least not now. Give it up for the present and get it off your mind best you can; that's because everything you say in your defense is most likely going to become something else they won't like about you or will argue with you about.

Perhaps later they'll see. Perhaps not. I can say that almost always, the children do come around.

Still, their opinions of you are not your prime issue now: Safety is your issue. Not their current thoughts.

As to defending yourself: When you say something and he comes back at you in an angry or critical way, it is normal, you are normal, to want to defend yourself. *He* is not normal!

He lives in a fantasy where he must be King and always right. Being always right is an important part of remaining King, you see. He has an unreal, abnormal (insane) take on the way things really are.

You just memorize "Yes Honey."

You do not have to mean it—only say it.

Practice it so often it just falls out of your mouth. Then Move Along.

* * *

About "Yes Honey"

Think of "Yes Honey" as a respectful (and safe) way to let him know you acknowledge his all-powerful, all-knowing self. This is the way it will come across most of the time too. It can be a haven of safety for you—your admiration or appreciation(even faked). You become less a target, safer because you are in his fan club.

If your efforts to be safe fail, you can likely save yourself from more even after a beating begins by telling him that you know he is right, and that you were wrong. Grovel. It sometimes works, though not instantly.

Then you must go for help as soon as ever you can. He will do it again. Don't lie to yourself about that.

Your life and the lives of your children or other family members can depend on your taking all of this very seriously— even if you think he isn't all that bad yet!

Any time his anger rises, especially when drinking or hungover, he is subject to lose what slim control he has on his emotions and behavior. You are almost always the nearest target; that's why his wrath explodes onto you—not because you actually did something he didn't like! It's because you're there. If it's the dog, he'll kick it. If it's a wall, he'll punch it.

After an angry explosion, an over-drinker has to justify what he has done; this means he will have worked the incident around in his head to where he comes out the good guy, or at least can blame someone else for causing him to do whatever he did.

He is defending his behavior and casting the blame for your black eye onto you! And when he tells others, they often buy it. Lord help us.

One woman's husband beat her for having so many bruises where they could be seen by others. She was ordered not to leave the house until the bruises healed. (I know; I was there.)

* * *

I remember: Fifty years ago, more than one policeman said to me, "You must like it; you went back!" They gave no thought to four small children that a woman with only a ninth-grade education must provide for. (In those days, the 1960s, she would not be able to rent a clean, safe apartment or buy a car without a man signing for her. Her wages were so low she had to work two jobs or rely on some man to bring in some money.

Survival back then for a woman with small children (which remains true to this day to a lesser extent) meant staying, going back, or going from man to man (most of whom fit the same profile as the first).

Yes, I did all the above.

* * *

Correcting the thinking of society by unremitting discussions and continuous publishing of facts can take years. It's already been 50 since my own experiences and we've come a long way—but not far enough. We're still not safe.

The purpose of this chapter has been to get you to reassess your situation, to rethink it.

Know this: The same number of women, or more, who died and were counted this year will die in this or the coming year. And the year after, and the year after that. . . .

This slaughter will continue until we educate every woman and girlchild about the dangers of being trapped in a relationship with such a man, and what to look for in a partner before they give their hearts away.

But, since most of *you* don't know very well how to do all that—yet, start looking for books to begin teaching you and other women who have come out successfully to teach you! And get involved in women's issues if you can.

An Ugly Truth

There is little evidence that an abuser ever overcomes his tendency to abuse, especially when he's drinking. Despite how sorry he says he is afterward (and he may really be terribly sorry), no matter how much he hates what he has done (and he probably does hate it), when he drinks again, he is very likely to do it again.

You can believe him when he says that he's sorry afterwards. You cannot believe him when he says he won't do it again.

Recognize that this man has almost no chance of getting better and begin searching for, reaching out for guidance and help. You can make trial calls to women's centers where other women give of themselves as volunteers. The woman answering the phone will likely also have experienced abuse and violence. They will give you support and information; they will totally understand you and your situation. They will even risk their own safety to go out and pick you up somewhere and take you to a safe place.

You can remain anonymous if you wish to talk to these incredible women, giving them only your first name. They aren't interested in your name, only your safety.

Two More Mottos

Bruising words do not come from a loving heart.

and

Sometimes love just ain't enough.

* * *

Well, My Lovelies! Our First Session Ends.

How I've enjoyed talking with you, giving you information not easily available, encouraging you I hope, giving you some tried and proved tools to work with to improve your life.

Hey—remember all those Mastery thoughts at the end of chapters? How about, once a week or once a month, go back over them. Repetition is how you build them into your everyday thinking.

This also is the time for you to look back at the list you made in the first chapter about what you wanted to get from this book. Look back there now and see if you did.

If we missed something, let us know! If you see any errors, or have questions, we would love to hear from you. I'll bet you're not the only one who would have liked to get that.. Contact me- us at www.hedrinkstoomuch.com

Join our blog; tune in and gradually begin to contribute your thinking and experience., add your comments, ask questions.

Get to know the thoughts of other women who are or have been in situations like yours. (Almost no one else will ever understand you completely.)

Now, I promised you that you would be changed after reading this book. Let me know if you are. Now you can teach other women these things. Scout around for a group. You can learn more there from others, and always share things you know that some others don't. The blog, too, is like a group, allowing you to communicate with women from all around the world— which is amazing! You can see others's stories, learn their thoughts and learn from their experiences.

I will answer your questions best I can on the blog, but I cannot give answers about specific situations or personalities. To do that safely requires knowing so many, many things about the person that I cannot possibly know without a therapeutic relationship. What I say to you might be just the wrong thing for another woman to take in.

I do though sometimes travel and hold workshops and do speaking and consulting. Perhaps we'll meet face to face some time in the future. I would love that!

And now, my lovely and oh-so-lovable princesses, so special, and for whom so many *good* men would joyously give their lives to care for,

I command you to do something daily that builds you up, and to start now gently caring for yourselves.

And start having more fun!

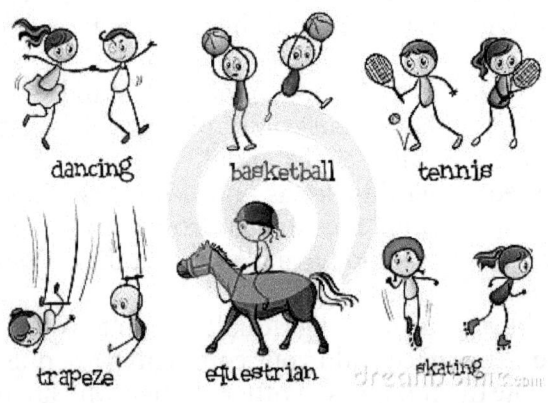

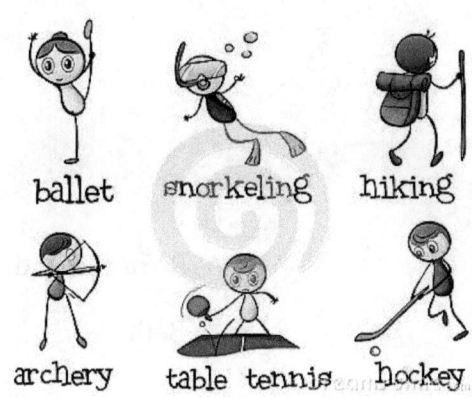

A N D
of course –

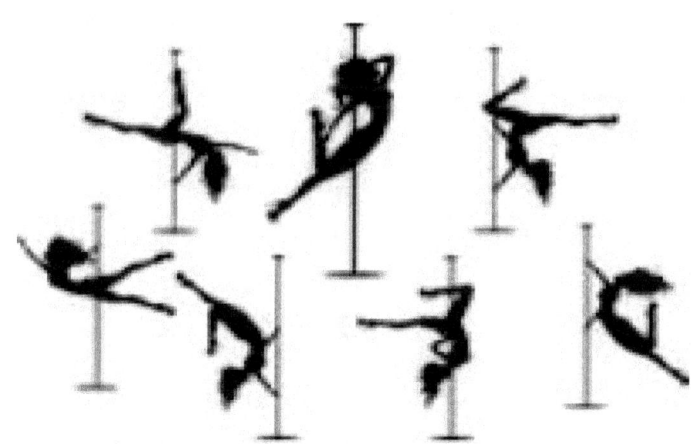

--ALWAYS Your Friend,

Beth

I'm nearly finished with Book 2 of this series, Curing Codependent Quirks. There's also a series "Fixin' My Picker, Psychology Meets Proverbs," Books 1 thru 5. (Our publisher currently handles phone calls for books as well as requests for workshops and speaking: Applied Psychology Publishing, LLC, in Jacksonville, Florida.)

www.hedrinkstoomuch.com

Join the conversation. Share your wisdom. Learn from others.

Note Pages

Note Pages

Note Pages

Note Pages

www.ingramcontent.com/pod-product-compliance
Lightning Source LLC
LaVergne TN
LVHW051109080426
835510LV00018B/1969